ROYAL HISTORICAL SOCIETY

STUDIES IN HISTORY

New Series

LEPROSY AND CHARITY
IN MEDIEVAL ROUEN

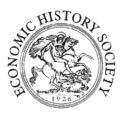

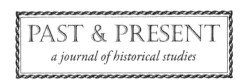

PAST & PRESENT
a journal of historical studies

LEPROSY AND CHARITY
IN MEDIEVAL ROUEN

Elma Brenner

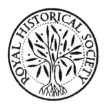

THE ROYAL HISTORICAL SOCIETY

THE BOYDELL PRESS

First published 2015

A Royal Historical Society publication
Published by The Boydell Press
an imprint of Boydell & Brewer Ltd
PO Box 9, Woodbridge, Suffolk IP12 3DF, UK
and of Boydell & Brewer Inc.
668 Mt Hope Avenue, Rochester, NY 14620–2731, USA
website: www.boydellandbrewer.com

ISBN 978–0–86193–339–6

ISSN 0269–2244

A CIP catalogue record for this book is available
from the British Library

The publisher has no responsibility for the continued existence or accuracy of
URLs for external or third-party internet websites referred to in this book,
and does not guarantee that any content on such websites is,
or will remain, accurate or appropriate

This publication is printed on acid-free paper

IN LOVING MEMORY
OF HEBA ZAMAN

Contents

Illustrations

Acknowledgements

A number of people and institutions deserve special thanks for helping me to bring this book to completion. Daniel Power, my advisor on the Editorial Board of the Royal Historical Society's *Studies in History* series, has encouraged me throughout the writing process, helped me to shape the structure of the book, and provided astute comments that improved the final manuscript. Elisabeth van Houts introduced me to the topic of leprosy and charity in medieval Rouen, and provided expert guidance as well as advising me on future projects. David Bates and Miri Rubin also made invaluable suggestions about the future directions of my research, and encouraged me to publish this monograph.

Much of the work for this book was completed during a Wellcome Trust Research Fellowship at the Department of History and Philosophy of Science at the University of Cambridge (2008–11). I am most grateful to the Wellcome Trust, the Department of History and Philosophy of Science, and Hughes Hall, where I had the privilege of being a Research Fellow between 2009 and 2011. I owe particular thanks to Peter Murray Jones, who sponsored my Wellcome Trust award. As an Andrew W. Mellon Post-Doctoral Fellow at the Pontifical Institute of Mediaeval Studies, University of Toronto, from 2011 to 2012, I benefited from a further period of research in a very stimulating and welcoming environment.

I am very grateful to the staff of the Archives départementales de Seine-Maritime, Rouen, and the Bibliothèque municipale, Rouen, for helping to make my archival research so profitable and enjoyable. I have also benefited from associate membership of the Centre de recherches archéologiques et historiques anciennes et médiévales, Université de Caen Basse-Normandie, since 2010, and have been able to make valuable use of the *Fonds normand* collection at the Université de Caen.

I thank Cath D'Alton for drawing the map, and Caroline Palmer for her advice and guidance. I am also most grateful to Christine Linehan for her excellent editorial work.

Completion of the book would not have been possible without the support of my family, friends and colleagues. I thank Marylin Brenner, Oswin Brenner, Salvador Alcántara Peláez and Jean Kirkley for all their support. Rachel Koopmans gave me invaluable advice about the structure of the book, and offered much encouragement. She is also owed thanks for granting me permission to reproduce Figure 1. Catherine Letouzey-Réty and Mickaël Réty were generous hosts in Rouen, and I benefited greatly from our discussions. I also warmly thank Richard Barnett, James Carley, Luke Demaitre, John Henderson, Leonie Hicks, Ann Hutchison, Fanny Madeline, †Diana

Parikian, Carole Rawcliffe, Bruno Tabuteau, François-Olivier Touati, Paul Webster and Emily Winkler. I am most grateful to my colleagues at the Wellcome Library since 2012, especially Richard Aspin, Elizabeth Graham and my other colleagues in the Special Collections and Research Department. This book is dedicated to the memory of my school friend Heba Zaman, who is dearly remembered and greatly missed.

Elma Brenner
September 2015

Abbreviations

ADSM   Archives départementales de Seine-Maritime, Rouen
AN   *Annales de Normandie*
AN, Paris   Archives nationales, Paris
ANS   *Anglo-Norman Studies*
BL   British Library, London
BM, Rouen   Bibliothèque municipale, Rouen
CTB   *The correspondence of Thomas Becket, archbishop of Canterbury,*
            1162–1170, ed. and trans. Anne J. Duggan, Oxford 2000
n.d.   undated
VCH   *Victoria County History*

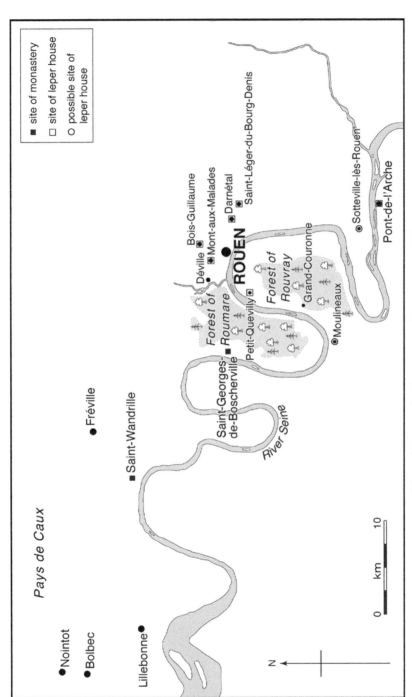

Upper Normandy, focusing on the environs of Rouen.

Introduction: Leprosy, Charity and Rouen

Leprosy has a prominent place in the modern-day imagination of the Middle Ages. There is much interest in how such a shocking disease, which has now disappeared from Western Europe, affected medieval society. The appearance of lepers in works of art, literature and miracle accounts, as well as the material remains of leper houses, testify to the contemporary cultural impact of the disease, despite the fact that only a very small proportion of the population actually contracted it. In the area around Rouen, one of the leading cities of medieval Western Europe, several *leprosaria* were established in the twelfth and thirteenth centuries, the most prominent being Mont-aux-Malades and Salle-aux-Puelles.[1] Leprosy and its sufferers had a distinctive impact on the society and religious culture of Rouen between the twelfth and fifteenth centuries. A detailed study of the city's leper houses thus sheds light on the social relationships and networks that shaped economic, political and devotional life in the city, and on changing responses to sickness and disease in this period. It also demonstrates the significant contribution made by the practice of charity, not only to provision for the sick and needy, but also to the forging of reciprocal bonds between different social groups.

Leprosy[2]

Responses to leprosy in medieval Europe were complex and often contradictory, reflecting the complicated moral and religious associations of the disease. Until the 1990s, scholarship tended to argue that lepers were socially excluded and stigmatised, and that leprosy was viewed as a punishment for sin.[3] In more recent decades, however, this viewpoint has been assessed critically, and has been traced back to the nineteenth century, when colonial encounters with lepers in extra-European settings influenced perspectives on medieval leprosy. It has been suggested that, instead, the leprous had

---

[1] The terms '*leprosarium*', 'leper house' and 'leper hospital' are used interchangeably in this book, to signify an organised institution that accommodated leprosy sufferers.

[2] This section is adapted from Elma Brenner, 'Recent perspectives on leprosy in medieval Western Europe', *History Compass* viii (2010), 388–406. I am grateful to Blackwell Publishing for permitting me to draw upon this article here.

[3] Proponents of this earlier view include Saul N. Brody, *The disease of the soul: leprosy in medieval literature*, Ithaca, NY 1974; R. I. Moore, *The formation of a persecuting society: power and deviance in Western Europe, 950–1250*, Oxford 1987; and Françoise Bériac, *Histoire des lépreux au moyen âge: une société d'exclus*, Paris 1988.

a special religious status in the Middle Ages, being believed to have been chosen by God to be redeemed, and were thus the objects of sympathy and compassion. Historians have also pointed towards the manners in which lepers were integrated, rather than segregated.[4] Admittedly, leper houses were almost always situated outside towns and cities, apparently following the biblical instruction that lepers should live 'without the camp' (Leviticus xiii.46). Yet these institutions remained connected to mainstream society as a key focus of charity, as well as through their economic activities as property-holders and centres of agricultural production.

Nonetheless, it is clear that in some instances lepers were overtly marginalised, and that concern about leprosy and contagion was a factor as early as the thirteenth century, becoming more widespread in the fourteenth. In the summer of 1321, lepers were accused of plotting to poison the waters of the kingdom of France, so that people would die or become leprous. The rumour was exploited by Philip v of France (1316–22), who on 21 June 1321 ordered that all lepers should be arrested, and those who confessed to the conspiracy be burned. In an atmosphere of heightened tension, many lepers were indeed burned to death. The Jews were also believed to be implicated in the conspiracy, and it was even suggested that the Muslim king of Granada was involved. The association of the leprous with Jews and Muslims in this rumour suggests that, at this particular point in time, they were viewed as outsiders. However, the persecution was short-lived, and occurred in the context of specific social and economic difficulties.[5] It was also restricted in geographical scope, mainly to southern and central France: there is no evidence that Rouen's lepers were persecuted in 1321. Chronicles from Rouen mention the violence, but do not refer to any persecution that took place specifically in the city.[6] Yet despite its limited impact, the 1321

---

[4] François-Olivier Touati spearheaded the re-thinking of responses to leprosy: 'Les Léproseries aux xIIème et xIIIème siècles, lieux de conversion?', in Nicole Bériou and François-Olivier Touati, *Voluntate dei leprosus: les lépreux entre conversion et exclusion aux XIIème et XIIIème siècles*, Spoleto 1991, 1–32; *Archives de la lèpre: atlas des léproseries entre Loire et Marne au moyen âge*, Paris 1996; and *Maladie et société au moyen âge: la lèpre, les lépreux et les léproseries dans la province ecclésiastique de Sens jusqu'au milieu du XIVe siècle*, Brussels 1998. Subsequently, Carole Rawcliffe and Luke Demaitre have made vital contributions: Carole Rawcliffe, *Leprosy in medieval England*, Woodbridge 2006; Luke Demaitre, *Leprosy in premodern medicine: a malady of the whole body*, Baltimore 2007.

[5] Malcolm Barber, 'Lepers, Jews and Moslems: the plot to overthrow Christendom in 1321', *History* lxvi (1981), 1–17, esp. pp. 1–7, 10–12. For an analysis of the 1321 crisis in a particular region, the Pays de Vaud (Switzerland), see Piera Borradori, *Mourir au monde: les lépreux dans le Pays de Vaud (XIIIe–XVIIe siècle)*, Lausanne 1992, 84–90.

[6] See 'E Chronici Rotomagensis continuatione', and 'E Chronico sanctæ Catharinæ de Monte Rothomagi', in *Recueil des historiens des Gaules et de la France*, xxiii, ed. J. N. de Wailly, L. V. Delisle and C. M. G. B. Jourdain, Paris 1876, 349, 409, and *Normanniae nova chronica ab anno Christi CCCCLXXIII. ad annum MCCCLXXVIII: e tribus chronicis mss. Sancti Laudi, Sanctae Catharinae et Majoris Ecclesiae Rotomagensium collecta*, ed. A. Chéruel, Caen 1850, 31.

persecution reflects the fact that, in the fourteenth century, less positive responses to the leprous, as well as the fear of contagion, started to replace the compassionate charity of the twelfth and thirteenth centuries.[7]

Leprosy is a bacterial infection that has two main forms, lepromatous leprosy and tuberculoid leprosy. The bacterium, *Mycobacterium leprae*, was identified in 1873 by G. H. Armauer Hansen, and the disease is now technically known as 'Hansen's disease'. Since both humans and diseases change biologically over time, it is difficult to know whether medieval leprosy took the same form as the modern strains of the disease.[8] However, some skeletal remains from medieval leper house cemeteries do provide evidence of the bone changes caused by Hansen's disease, at least in its advanced lepromatous form. This type of leprosy, probably the dominant form in the past, is manifested in large skin sores, and, ultimately, degeneration of the facial features, particularly the nose and palate, and destruction of the nerves at the bodily extremities, such as the fingers and toes, resulting in loss of sensation and thus damage to these areas (*see* Figure 1).[9] Archaeologists in England, France and Denmark have excavated skeletons affected by these changes to the bones of the face, hands and feet.[10] At the cemetery of the leper house of St James and St Mary Magdalene, Chichester, for example, at least seventy-five of 384 skeletons excavated showed bone changes, with thirty-seven exhibiting damage to the bones of the face.[11] Like the lepromatous form, tuberculoid leprosy results in loss of sensation, as well as weakened muscles. However, it tends to be less long lasting than lepromatous leprosy,

---

[7] See Barber, 'Lepers, Jews and Moslems', 14–15.

[8] Jesper L. Boldsen, 'Epidemiological approach to the paleopathological diagnosis of leprosy', *American Journal of Physical Anthropology* cxv (2001), 380.

[9] Harvey Marcovitch (ed.), *Black's medical dictionary*, 41st edn, London 2005, 406; Frances Lee and Keith Manchester, 'Leprosy: a review of the evidence in the Chichester sample', in John Magilton, Frances Lee and Anthea Boylston (eds), *'Lepers outside the gate': excavations at the cemetery of the hospital of St James and St Mary Magdalene, Chichester, 1986–87 and 1993*, York 2008, 209; Peter Richards, *The medieval leper and his northern heirs*, Cambridge 1977, repr. 2000, pp. xv, xvi; Carole Rawcliffe, 'Learning to love the leper: aspects of institutional charity in Anglo-Norman England', ANS xxiii (2000), 232; David Marcombe, *Leper knights: the Order of St Lazarus of Jerusalem in England, 1150–1544*, Woodbridge 2003, 135–6.

[10] Simon Roffey, 'Medieval leper hospitals in England: an archaeological perspective', *Medieval Archaeology* lvi (2012), 216–17. See, for example, findings at Chichester (Magilton, Lee and Boylston, *'Lepers outside the gate'*), Aizier (Cécile Niel and Marie-Cécile Truc [with Bruno Penna], 'La Chapelle Saint-Thomas d'Aizier (Eure): premiers résultats de six années de fouille programmée', in Bruno Tabuteau [ed.], *Étude des lépreux et des léproseries au moyen âge dans le nord de la France: histoire – archéologie – patrimoine*, Histoire Médiévale et Archéologie xx [2007], 47–107) and Naestved, Denmark (Richards, *The medieval leper*, 116–18).

[11] Frances Lee and John Magilton, 'Discussion', in Magilton, Lee and Boylston, *'Lepers outside the gate'*, 265–6.

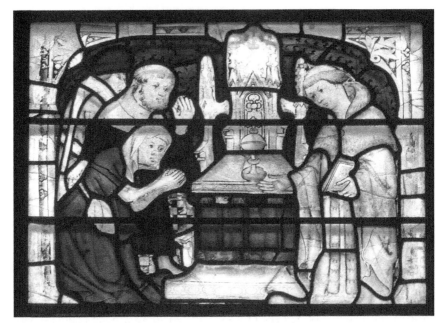

Figure 1. A leprous woman (below left) kneeling to pray before the shrine of St William, in a fifteenth-century stained glass panel at York Minster, England. This is part of the St William window, which shows miraculous events associated with the saint's shrine and tomb. Sores are visible on the woman's face, and her thin arms suggest that she is frail.

and does not leave such visible traces in skeletal remains.[12] Lepromatous leprosy has additional debilitating symptoms that are not reflected in the bones of sufferers, particularly damaged vocal capacity, breathing problems and blindness. The disease can thus cause severe impairment and disfigurement, with which sufferers often live for a number of years. It is now held that leprosy is not heavily contagious, although the manner of transmission is still not fully understood.[13]

The religious status of lepers is a key issue. François-Olivier Touati argues that *leprosaria*, as monastic institutions, were intended to serve as sites for the conversion of lepers to the religious life. The theologian Peter of Poitiers (d. 1215) placed lepers in the category of the religious, and suggested that they should renounce the world and live in obedience to a religious rule.

---

[12] Lee and Manchester, 'Leprosy: a review of the evidence', 208; Roffey, 'Medieval leper hospitals', 216.

[13] *Black's medical dictionary*, 406; François-Olivier Touati, 'Contagion and leprosy: myth, ideas and evolution in medieval minds and societies', in Lawrence I. Conrad and Dominik Wujastyk (eds), *Contagion: perspectives from pre-modern societies*, Aldershot 2000, 179.

This process entailed the fulfilment of penance and a religious conversion.[14] The numerous benefactions to *leprosaria* in the twelfth and thirteenth centuries may be explained by a wish to support lepers in pursuing a religious vocation, and by the fact that the prayers of lepers, who were among God's elect, were seen to be particularly efficacious in bringing about the donor's salvation.[15]

In his conception of the structure of society, the French theologian Jacques de Vitry (d. 1240) categorised lepers with other sick people. According to de Vitry, the Church consisted of thirty different *status*, which he placed in order according to their various states of perfection. The religious preceded the laity in this hierarchy: clerics were placed first, followed by monks and all those who lived in fraternities, including hospital communities. Although (unlike in Peter of Poitiers's scheme) lepers were placed among the laity, they and other sick persons occupied the highest category of this group, which also included the poor, the grieving, pilgrims and those who had taken the cross. Since these people were understood to be being tested by God, they were considered spiritually superior to the rest of the laity.[16] Nicole Bériou argues that the manner in which de Vitry addressed 'lepers and the other sick' in his sermons indicates that he considered lepers to be representative of the sick in general.[17]

Leprosaria, where lepers were often members of a religious community, are one of the primary sources of evidence about the disease and its sufferers in medieval Western Europe. This book's study of Rouen's leper houses sits alongside studies of institutions for lepers in other parts of Upper Normandy, at Pont-Audemer, Évreux and Aizier.[18] It is also informed by work on *leprosaria* in other regions, including England, Ireland, Catalonia, the Pays de Vaud region of Switzerland and the Pas-de-Calais area of northern France.[19]

---

[14] Touati, 'Les Léproseries aux XIIème et XIIIème siècles?', 3–19.

[15] See Rawcliffe, *Leprosy*, 142.

[16] Nicole Bériou, 'Les Lépreux sous le regard des prédicateurs d'après les collections de sermons *ad status* du XIIIème siècle', in Bériou and Touati, *Voluntate dei leprosus*, 39–40.

[17] 'les lépreux et les autres malades': ibid. 41.

[18] On the leper house at Pont-Audemer see Simone C. Mesmin, 'The leper hospital of Saint Gilles de Pont-Audemer: an edition of its cartulary and an examination of the problem of leprosy in the twelfth and early thirteenth century', unpubl. PhD diss. Reading 1978; 'Waleran, count of Meulan and the leper hospital of S. Gilles de Pont-Audemer', AN xxxii (1982), 3–19; and 'Du Comte à la commune: la léproserie de Saint-Gilles de Pont-Audemer', AN xxxvii (1987), 235–67. On the leper house at Évreux see Bruno Tabuteau, 'Une Léproserie normande au moyen âge: le prieuré de Saint-Nicolas d'Évreux du XIIe au XVIe siècle: histoire et corpus des sources', unpubl. PhD diss. Rouen 1996. On the leper house at Aizier see Niel and Truc, 'La Chapelle Saint-Thomas d'Aizier'.

[19] Rawcliffe, *Leprosy*; Max Satchell, 'The emergence of leper-houses in medieval England, 1100–1250', unpubl. D.Phil diss. Oxford 1998; Gerard A. Lee, *Leper hospitals in medieval Ireland: with a short account of the military and Hospitaller order of St Lazarus*

Above all, these studies have demonstrated that, for a number of reasons, leper houses retained links with mainstream society. Indeed, they were often situated along main roads and sometimes located close to city gates, making them highly visible.[20] *Leprosaria* were also connected to the world by virtue of their role as a major focus of charity. Canon 23 of the Third Lateran Council of 1179 provided for every group of lepers to have its own church, cemetery and priest, confirming that leper houses were religious institutions.[21] They could thus be categorised with other religious houses as worthy destinations for charity, and offered the opportunity for benefactors to obtain the powerful intercessory prayers of lepers on behalf of their souls.

Charity

Charity, the highest Christian virtue, is defined in the Bible as love of God and love of one's neighbour, urging both pious and practical activities (1 Corinthians xiii.13; 1 John iv.21). The Bible also outlines six corporal works of mercy: feeding the hungry, giving drink to the thirsty, granting hospitality to strangers, clothing the naked, visiting the sick, and visiting prisoners. A seventh, the burial of the dead, was added in the course of the Middle Ages. At the Last Judgement, Christ admits to heaven only those who have fulfilled these works (Matthew xxv.31–46). Medieval Christians were highly aware of the need to fulfil the works of mercy to ensure the future salvation of their souls, and did so literally (for example, by visiting prisoners, by making donations on behalf of the needy, or by praying on their behalf). Charity was a mutually beneficial and reciprocal process, since benefactors were thereby able to amass spiritual credit for their souls, enhanced by the prayers that they expected to receive from those whom they assisted. Benefactors could also strengthen their reputation in worldly society by displaying their generosity and sense of social responsibility. Charity was already an essential aspect of religious culture in the twelfth century, as chapter 1, surveying the early endowment of the leper house of Mont-aux-Malades at Rouen, demonstrates. In the twelfth and thirteenth centuries, responding to

of Jerusalem, Blackrock, Co. Dublin 1996; James W. Brodman, 'Shelter and segregation: lepers in medieval Catalonia', in Donald J. Kagay and Theresa M. Vann (eds), *On the social origins of medieval institutions: essays in honor of Joseph F. O'Callaghan*, Leiden 1998, 35–45; Borradori, *Mourir au monde*; Albert Bourgeois, *Lépreux et maladreries du Pas-de-Calais (Xe–XVIIIe siècles)*, Arras 1972.

20 On the topography of *leprosaria* see François-Olivier Touati, 'La Géographie hospitalière médiévale (Orient–Occident, IVe–XVIe siècles): des modèles aux réalités', in Pascal Montaubin (ed.), *Hôpitaux et maladreries au moyen âge: espace et environnement*, Histoire Médiévale et Archéologie xvii (2004), 7–20.

21 *Decrees of the ecumenical councils*, ed. and trans. Norman P. Tanner, London 1990, i. 222–3; Jean Avril, 'Le IIIe Concile du Latran et les communautés de lépreux', *Revue Mabillon* lx (1981), 21–76.

the idea of Purgatory, a doctrine formalised at the Second Council of Lyon in 1274, Christians exhibited considerable concern about the future fate of their souls and about ensuring that the living would continue to pray for them after death.[22] The heightened engagement in charitable works in the thirteenth century was also linked to broader changes in practices of piety at this time, such as the foundation of private masses in chantry chapels and the establishment of lights at altars.[23]

There was also a broader social and economic context for the growth of charity. Before the Black Death, there was significant population increase and urban expansion in Western Europe, which caused an increase in the numbers of wandering poor. As society became increasingly mercantile, those making large sums of money began to question the morality of their profit-making activities.[24] Many of the wealthier members of society chose to distribute their surplus income to the needy.[25] Such actions could also be governed by self-interest: some Italian merchants engaged in usury, for example, elected to fulfil charitable works rather than make restitution for interest that they had exacted illegally.[26]

Religious and intellectual trends in the twelfth and thirteenth centuries were also crucial to the emergence of practices of charity. Theologians began to distinguish between voluntary and involuntary poverty. While the voluntary poor were members of monastic communities, who had chosen to retreat from the world, the involuntary poor were those who suffered a physical or material need through no choice of their own. In the last part of the twelfth century, the latter group became known as the 'poor of Christ' (previously, the 'poor of Christ' had signified the voluntary poor). At the University of Paris in the late twelfth century, Peter the Chanter and his followers discussed the obligations of the Christian community to the poor and promoted the active over the contemplative life, thus encouraging the practical activities involved in fulfilling charitable works. Twelfth- and thirteenth-century canon lawyers were also interested in the issue of poverty, and argued that the poor should not be deprived of their legal rights. Indeed, by the beginning of the thirteenth century, it was understood that the poor

---

[22] See Mailan S. Doquang, 'Status and the soul: commemoration and intercession in the Rayonnant chapels of northern France in the thirteenth and fourteenth centuries', in Elma Brenner, Meredith Cohen and Mary Franklin-Brown (eds), *Memory and commemoration in medieval culture*, Farnham 2013, 97–9.

[23] On chantry chapels see ibid. 93–9; on lights see David Postles, 'Lamps, lights and layfolk: "popular" devotion before the Black Death', *Journal of Medieval History* xxv (1999), 97–114.

[24] James W. Brodman, *Charity and religion in medieval Europe*, Washington, DC 2009, 14–15.

[25] Bronislaw Geremek, *Poverty: a history*, trans. A. Kolakowska, Oxford 1994, 22, 23; Lester K. Little, *Religious poverty and the profit economy in medieval Europe*, London 1978, pp. vii, ix–x, 211–13.

[26] Little, *Religious poverty*, 211–13.

had a right to material assistance from the Church and from those people who had surplus wealth.[27] The growth of the mendicant orders, members of which themselves embraced a life of voluntary poverty, enhanced this emphasis on the needs and entitlements of the poor. It is noteworthy that the Franciscan archbishop of Rouen, Eudes Rigaud (1248–75), took steps to establish a *leprosarium* on his manor at Aliermont in the mid-thirteenth century, and consistently took an interest in hospitals and leper houses during his rounds of visitation.[28]

By the thirteenth century, charitable benefactors distinguished between those whom they considered deserving and those undeserving of receiving assistance. Broadly speaking, the 'true' ('deserving') poor were sick, disabled, orphaned, elderly or widowed, while the 'false' ('undeserving') poor were idle beggars who were capable of working but did not seek employment.[29] In late medieval Florence, for example, the 'shame-faced poor' ('poveri vergognosi'), those who had fallen from a respectable position in society and were embarrassed to beg, were deemed to be the worthy recipients of the charity offered by confraternities.[30] Canon lawyers were instrumental in defining these different categories of the needy. Gratian stated that the distribution of charity should prioritise friends, the humble and the honest.[31] Raymond of Penyafort (c.1175–1275) similarly argued that, where resources were limited, family and friends should be favoured. The charitable practices of confraternities, which placed the needs of confraternity members first, clearly followed this model. Canon lawyers also argued that almsgiving should be directed more towards the sick than the healthy.[32] The prayers of the deserving needy were perceived to be much more efficacious than those of the undeserving, as well as more reliable. Lepers, at least to those who saw them as a group chosen by God to suffer on earth and be saved, formed an exemplary category of the deserving needy.

Much of the support for medieval *leprosaria* also fits into broader patterns of monastic patronage. Many larger institutions for lepers were organised as religious communities following a rule, and might be one of a number of religious houses to which individuals and families offered benefaction.

---

[27] Brodman, *Charity and religion*, 15–19.

[28] See appendix 2, no. 19(a); *Regestrum visitationum archiepiscopi Rothomagensis: journal des visites pastorales d'Eude Rigaud, archevêque de Rouen, MCCXLVIII–MCCLXIX*, ed. Théodose Bonnin, Rouen 1852; *The Register of Eudes of Rouen*, trans. Sydney M. Brown and ed. Jeremiah F. O'Sullivan, New York 1964.

[29] Bronislaw Geremek, *The margins of society in late medieval Paris*, trans. J. Birrell, Cambridge 1987, 169; Michel Mollat, *Les Pauvres au moyen âge: étude sociale*, Paris 1978, 12, 17–18.

[30] John Henderson, *Piety and charity in late medieval Florence*, Oxford 1994, 36, 149, 255–6, 373.

[31] Brodman, *Charity and religion*, 29.

[32] Ibid.

Charitable transactions were connected both to the desire of lay patrons to procure their salvation, and to the status of monastic houses as major holders of land and property, necessitating negotiation and agreement between religious and laity. The relationship formed between benefactor and recipient continued from one generation to the next, although it was reshaped over time.[33] Like hospitals for the sick poor, many leper house communities followed the Augustinian rule, which underlined the need to provide for the sick.[34] This order, observed by regular canons, was a major focus of religious patronage in Normandy in the twelfth and thirteenth centuries, from the end of Henry I's reign onwards.[35] The Augustinians were actively involved in lay society, tending the sick, distributing alms and supporting parish communities. At the same time, the regular life provided opportunities for lay people to live alongside Augustinian canons in service to the poor and sick.[36] A number of charitable institutions, such as the leper house at Bois-Halbout (*département* of Calvados), founded between 1165 and 1171 by the layman Robert fitz Erneis and subsequently managed by the Augustinian canons of Notre-Dame-du-Val, developed as a result of a close collaboration between Augustinian communities and members of the laity.[37]

The fervour for charity of the twelfth and thirteenth centuries, which led to the establishment of numerous hospitals and *leprosaria* in Western Europe, was not sustained in the later Middle Ages. In many regions the troubles of the fourteenth century, which witnessed famines, the arrival of the plague and protracted periods of warfare, meant that groups who had previously supported the poor and sick were themselves in need of assistance. Furthermore, the social dislocation caused by these events resulted in growing numbers of the wandering poor, who were excluded from the provision offered by local networks such as confraternities and parishes, and were associated with crime and the spread of disease.[38] Charity thus became

[33] See Emilia Jamroziak, *Rievaulx abbey and its social context, 1132–1300: memory, locality, and networks*, Turnhout 2005, 57–61.

[34] 'The Rule of Augustine (masculine version)', in *The Rule of Saint Augustine*, ed. Tarsicius J. van Bavel and trans. Raymond Canning, Kalamazoo 1996, 15, 21.

[35] For Augustinian hospitals and leper houses in Normandy see Mathieu Arnoux, 'Les Origines et le développement du mouvement canonial en Normandie', in Mathieu Arnoux (ed.), *Des Clercs au service de la réforme: études et documents sur les chanoines réguliers de la province de Rouen*, Turnhout 2000, 119–27.

[36] Leonie V. Hicks, *Religious life in Normandy, 1050–1300: space, gender and social pressure*, Woodbridge 2007, 7, 17, 62–4; François-Olivier Touati, '"Aime et fais ce que tu veux": les chanoines réguliers et la revolution de charité au moyen âge', in Michel Parisse (ed.), *Les Chanoines réguliers: émergence et expansion (XIe–XIIIe siècle); actes du sixième colloque international du CERCOR, Le Puy en Velay, 29 juin–1er juillet 2006*, Saint-Étienne 2009, 159–210.

[37] Touati, '"Aime et fais ce que tu veux"', 205–6; Hicks, *Religious life*, 205.

[38] On these issues in one region, Catalonia, see James W. Brodman, *Charity and welfare: hospitals and the poor in medieval Catalonia*, Philadelphia 1998, 138–43.

increasingly discriminating, and the support received by leper houses and hospitals was reduced. As one of the major cities of medieval Europe, Rouen experienced many of these changes, as the foci and distribution of charitable aid shifted between the twelfth and fifteenth centuries.

Rouen

The chief city of Normandy in the central and later Middle Ages, Rouen was a leading political, ecclesiastical and trading centre. Although a wide-ranging collection of essays has recently been published on the medieval city, much remains to be discovered from the rich documentary and material evidence from Rouen.[39] The twelfth and thirteenth centuries in particular marked a pivotal period in the city's history, which witnessed the emergence of a dominant burgess elite, Rouen's annexation to France in 1204, and major topographical and commercial growth. Rouen was a Norman 'capital' on a par with Paris in this period.[40] The city experienced a period of turbulence and decline in the fourteenth and fifteenth centuries, due to the upheaval caused by the Hundred Years' War (1337–1453), as well as the impact of the Black Death of 1348 and subsequent plague outbreaks. Changing responses to leprosy and its sufferers, and changes in practices of charity, therefore need to be seen in the context of the social and economic crises of the later Middle Ages.

In the first part of the twelfth century, the chronicler Orderic Vitalis described Rouen as 'A populous and wealthy city, thronged with merchants and a meeting-place of trade routes.' He emphasised Rouen's beauty, abundant natural resources and strong fortifications.[41] In Orderic's *Ecclesiastical history*, it is claimed that, in 1090, the future King Henry I stated that Rouen 'has rightly been the capital of all Normandy from the earliest days'.[42] The most visible aspect of the city's eleventh- and twelfth-century growth was its

---

[39] Leonie V. Hicks and Elma Brenner (eds), *Society and culture in medieval Rouen, 911–1300*, Turnhout 2013. See also Jenny Stratford (ed.), *Medieval art, architecture and archaeology at Rouen*, [London] 1993; Michel Mollat (ed.), *Histoire de Rouen*, Toulouse 1979.

[40] See David Bates, 'Rouen from 900 to 1204: from Scandinavian settlement to Angevin "capital"', in Stratford, *Medieval art, architecture and archaeology*, 1, 5; Bernard Gauthiez, 'Paris, un Rouen capétien? (Développements comparés de Rouen et Paris sous les règnes de Henri II et Philippe Auguste)', ANS xvi (1993), 117, 119, 121, 123, and 'The urban development of Rouen, 989–1345', in Hicks and Brenner, *Society and culture*, 34.

[41] 'Rodomensis ciuitas populis est ac negociorum commerciis opulentissima, portus quoque confluentia': *The ecclesiastical history of Orderic Vitalis*, ed. and trans. Marjorie Chibnall, Oxford 1969–80, iii. 36–7; Bates, 'Rouen', 1; Lucien Musset, 'Rouen au temps des Francs et sous les ducs (ve siècle–1204)', in Mollat, *Histoire de Rouen*, 53.

[42] 'cui iure a priscis temporibus subiacet Normannia tota': *Ecclesiastical history of Orderic Vitalis*, iv. 224–5; Bates, 'Rouen', 1; Musset, 'Rouen', 53–4.

topographical expansion. New religious houses and other architectural works also reflected significant development. A new wall built between 1067 and 1090 encompassed an area of expansion to the west of the city.[43] By the early twelfth century, there was already continuous settlement from the walled city to the suburban area outside, since in 1116 a fire spread beyond the city walls.[44] New walls built under Henry II, possibly between 1150 and 1160, incorporated the Benedictine abbey of Saint-Ouen, previously located in the suburbs. By the early thirteenth century, three new parishes had emerged in the newly enclosed area, Saint-Patrice, Saint-Godard and Saint-Maclou.[45] Thus, the urban zone was redefined as a much larger entity.

While Saint-Ouen was a Merovingian foundation, several new religious houses were established in the eleventh century, among them the abbey of La Trinité-du-Mont and its sister house of Saint-Amand, founded by Goscelin, son of Heddon, *vicomte* of Arques and his wife Emmeline in about 1035–40, the priory of Notre-Dame du Pré, established by William the Conqueror's wife Matilda of Flanders around 1060, and the priories of Saint-Gervais and Saint-Paul.[46] All were located in the suburbs, reflecting the city's steady expansion. Within the walls, a hospital for the sick, the Hôtel-Dieu, was built in the eleventh century or possibly earlier. It was probably founded by the archbishop and cathedral chapter, and building work may have been carried out in conjunction with work on the Romanesque cathedral, dedicated in 1063.[47]

The twelfth century saw a number of Augustinian foundations. The leper house of Mont-aux-Malades was established in the early twelfth century to the north-west of Rouen, and was under the management of Augustinian canons by the reign of Henry II, if not earlier. The Augustinian priory of La Madeleine, a community of canons and lay sisters and brothers, was established in about 1154 to oversee the Hôtel-Dieu, henceforth known as La Madeleine hospital.[48] The priory of Saint-Lô, which had previously been

---

[43] Gauthiez, 'Urban development', 28–30.

[44] Musset, 'Rouen', 54.

[45] Gauthiez, 'Paris, un Rouen capétien?', 119; Bates, 'Rouen', 2; Gauthiez, 'Urban development', 30–1.

[46] Musset, 'Rouen', 48, 53, 58; François Burckard, *Guide des archives de la Seine-Maritime*, I: *Généralités; archives antérieures à 1790*, Rouen 1990, 391, 397, 410–11; Bates, 'Rouen', 4; Kirsten A. Fenton, 'Women, property, and power: some examples from eleventh-century Rouen cartularies', in Hicks and Brenner, *Society and culture*, 235 (foundation of La Trinité-du-Mont), 236–7 (early donations to Saint-Amand).

[47] Burckard, *Guide*, 423; Marc Boulanger, *Les Hôpitaux de Rouen: une longue et attachante histoire: des origines à nos jours*, Luneray 1988, 17; Musset, 'Rouen', 73.

[48] Musset, 'Rouen', 58; Boulanger, *Les Hôpitaux*, 17–18. On La Madeleine see also Louis Rousseau, 'L'Assistance charitable à Rouen du XIIe au XVIe siècle: l'Hôtel-Dieu de la Madeleine: la police des pauvres', unpubl. thesis, École nationale des Chartes, Paris 1938, and Elma Brenner, 'The care of the sick and needy in twelfth- and thirteenth-century Rouen', in Hicks and Brenner, *Society and culture*, 344.

the seat of the exiled bishop and chapter of Coutances, was transformed into an Augustinian community in 1144.[49] The *leprosarium* of Salle-aux-Puelles, which provided for high-status leprous women, was organised as a priory headed by a prior and a prioress by the mid-thirteenth century, although no information survives about the rule that this community followed.

Henry II was particularly responsible for major developments at Rouen in the second half of the twelfth century. His parents, Geoffrey, count of Anjou (1129–51) and duke of Normandy (1145–50), and the Empress Matilda, had already begun to develop the city's infrastructure. Geoffrey built a wooden bridge across the Seine that subsequently burned down; Matilda paid for the construction of the first stone bridge, built between 1151 and 1167.[50] In the late 1150s building works were also carried out at Quevilly, on the other side of the Seine, where Henry I had built a new ducal residence.[51] The Saint-Romain tower was added to Rouen cathedral in the 1160s, and the main roads of the city were probably paved before 1200. In addition to the expansion represented by Henry II's new walls on the right bank of the Seine, on the left bank the area south of the church of Saint-Sever was settled by the early thirteenth century. These changes testify to Rouen's growing population and prosperity, and its increasingly urbanised appearance in the late twelfth and thirteenth centuries.[52]

The basis of Rouen's expansion was its commercial success, derived from its strategic position on the river Seine. By the twelfth century, Rouen had several long-established trading links, above all with England and Ireland.[53] The city also developed more distant connections: early in the eleventh century, Dudo of Saint-Quentin included Frisians, Greeks, Danes and Indians among its visitors.[54] Rouen was a point of exchange for products from other areas of Normandy, and in particular for the transportation of salt and fish to Paris. Above all, however, its commerce was based on wine. The banks of the Seine were lined with wine cellars, many of which were privately owned by religious houses and leading burgesses. The wine trade, which supplied London and other parts of southern and eastern England, was

---

[49] Arnoux, 'Les Origines', 21, 64–9; François Lemoine and Jacques Tanguy, *Rouen aux 100 clochers: dictionnaire des églises et chapelles de Rouen (avant 1789)*, Rouen 2004, 119; Musset, 'Rouen', 57, 58.

[50] Fanny Madeline, 'Rouen and its place in the building policy of the Angevin kings', in Hicks and Brenner, *Society and culture*, 73; Musset, 'Rouen', 56; Bates, 'Rouen', 5; Gauthiez, 'Paris, un Rouen capétien?', 119; *Chronique de Robert de Torigni, abbé du Mont-Saint-Michel*, ed. Léopold Delisle, Rouen 1872–3, i. 239, 368.

[51] Gauthiez, 'Paris, un Rouen capétien?', 119; Bates, 'Rouen', 4. On the manor at Quevilly and other building works by Henry II in the area around Rouen see Madeline, 'Rouen and its place', 68–71.

[52] Gauthiez, 'Paris, un Rouen capétien?', 119, 121.

[53] Musset, 'Rouen', 70–1; Bates, 'Rouen', 6.

[54] Bates, 'Rouen', 1.

badly affected by the separation of Normandy from England in 1204, when London's citizens began to trade with the wine merchants of La Rochelle and, later, Bordeaux.[55]

Although the Norman Exchequer was located at Caen from the reign of Henry II, Rouen was one of the major financial centres of the Anglo-Norman realm. In the twelfth and thirteenth centuries, the financial district was focused around the church of Notre-Dame de la Ronde and along the rue du Gros-Horloge, immediately west of the cathedral. Rouen's Jewish quarter was directly adjacent to this area, underlining the prominence of the Jews in financial affairs, particularly in lending large sums to the king and leading citizens.[56]

The merchant elite of Rouen, which included a handful of converted Jews among its number, gained a large degree of political autonomy during the second half of the twelfth century.[57] Henry II granted a 'charter of liberties' to the citizens of Rouen in about 1150–1 (as duke of Normandy, before acceding to the English throne in 1154), according them judicial protection, the right to consent to ducal taxation and full control over trade at Rouen.[58] These customs may have dated back to the reign of Henry I. Between 1160 and 1170 they were incorporated in the *Établissements de Rouen*, a document that marks the existence of the commune, or municipal government, of Rouen. The *Établissements* describes the organisation of the commune, which was composed of 100 citizens (*pairs*) who met every fifteen days and had a primarily judicial role. The mayor, whose office was made annually renewable when the *Établissements* was modified in 1204, had substantial military, financial and judicial powers, although the king retained the power of high justice and the right to appoint the mayor. Twelve councillors (*conseillers*) and twelve aldermen (*échevins*) assisted the mayor.[59]

Communal offices were filled by the merchants, whose growing prosperity is evidenced by the construction of a stone market hall near the main market square, the *Vieux Marché*, by about 1186, and its enlargement in 1192.[60] This patriciate, composed of leading families such as the Du Châtel, the

---

[55] Ibid. 6; Musset, 'Rouen', 69–70.

[56] Gauthiez, 'Paris, un Rouen capétien?', 123, 127; Norman Golb, *Les Juifs de Rouen au moyen âge: portrait d'une culture oubliée*, Rouen 1985, 3–30, 101–42; Elma Brenner and Leonie V. Hicks, 'The Jews of Rouen in the eleventh to the thirteenth centuries', in Hicks and Brenner, *Society and culture*, 369, 376.

[57] Brenner and Hicks, 'The Jews of Rouen', 378–9.

[58] *Regesta regum Anglo-Normannorum, 1066–1154*, ed. H. A. Cronne, R. H. C. Davis and others, Oxford 1913–69, iii. 268–9 (no. 729); Bates, 'Rouen', 5; Musset, 'Rouen', 61.

[59] Musset, 'Rouen', 61–3; A. Giry, *Les Établissements de Rouen: études sur l'histoire des institutions municipales de Rouen, Falaise, Pont-Audemer, etc.*, Paris 1883–5, i. 14–20.

[60] Musset, 'Rouen', 69; Gauthiez, 'Paris, un Rouen capétien?', 123; Daniel Power, 'Angevin Normandy', in Christopher Harper-Bill and Elisabeth van Houts (eds), *A companion to the Anglo-Norman world*, Woodbridge 2003, 81.

Val-Richer, the Le Gros and the Le Changeur, was not shaken from its dominant position by the new political situation after 1204.[61] The *Établissements* was a very influential document, providing a model for municipal governments elsewhere in Normandy and western France. By 1204 communes had been instituted in every major Norman town except Lisieux; the organisation of towns such as Pont-Audemer and Falaise directly followed that of Rouen.[62]

While the burgesses dominated Rouen's communal government, the Anglo-Norman aristocracy also played a significant role in the city, attending assemblies, supplying canons to the cathedral chapter, and endowing monastic houses, including leper houses and hospitals. Certain aristocratic lineages, such as the counts of Eu, the counts of Leicester and the Marshal earls of Pembroke, were major property-holders in the city.[63] Some of these landed interests, such as those of the Marshal earls, were retained after 1204, although many Anglo-Norman noble families retreated from Rouen after Philip Augustus took control of the city.[64]

Normandy's annexation to the French royal domain in 1204 had a significant impact on Rouen's political and commercial status, but the city continued to develop in the thirteenth century.[65] Commerce with England was undoubtedly hampered by political difficulties after 1204. Although Philip Augustus of France (1180–1223) and John of England (1199–1216) concluded a truce in 1214, it was broken three times before 1250, and during these periods Rouen merchants trading in England had to acquire safe conducts to protect themselves from imprisonment and the confiscation of their goods. However, the situation greatly improved after the mid-thirteenth century. In addition, Rouen's economy was bolstered by cloth production, an industry which developed from the late twelfth century. In the thirteenth century, high quality wool began to be imported from England, and Rouen merchants travelled to fairs in France and Italy to sell their cloth.[66]

---

[61] Musset, 'Rouen', 64; Suzanne Deck, 'Les Marchands de Rouen sous les ducs', AN vi (1956), 249. On Rouen's burgesses see also Manon Six, 'The burgesses of Rouen in the late twelfth and early thirteenth centuries', in Hicks and Brenner, *Society and culture*, 247–78; Alain Sadourny, 'Les Grandes Familles rouennaises au XIIIe siècle et leur rôle dans la cité', in Pierre Bouet and François Neveux (eds), *Les Villes normandes au moyen âge: renaissance, essor, crise: actes du colloque international de Cerisy-la-Salle (8–12 octobre 2003)*, Caen 2006, 267–78.

[62] Musset, 'Rouen', 61; Bates, 'Rouen', 5; Power, 'Angevin Normandy', 82.

[63] Daniel Power, 'Rouen and the aristocracy of Angevin Normandy', in Hicks and Brenner, *Society and culture*, 283–5, 288–9.

[64] See pp. 38–9 below for discussion of Richard Marshal's Norman interests in the 1220s.

[65] For the general situation in Normandy after 1204 see Daniel Power, *The Norman frontier in the twelfth and early thirteenth centuries*, Cambridge 2004, ch. xiii.

[66] Alain Sadourny, 'L'Époque communale (1204–début du XIVe siècle)', in Mollat, *Histoire de Rouen*, 77–8, 81–3.

Rouen's burgess community continued to dominate civic affairs in the thirteenth century. In 1207 Philip Augustus issued a charter confirming the city's privileges, which reiterated the earlier acts of the dukes of Normandy, and confirmed the commercial and judicial powers of the commune. In particular, Rouen's citizens retained their monopoly of trade on the lower Seine, and were entrusted with powers of justice relating to civil and commercial affairs. The charter remained the definitive text of Rouen's privileges for the next 150 years.[67] Many burgesses profited from the new cloth industry: the Val-Richer family, for example, which contributed eight mayors to Rouen in the thirteenth century, owned most of the cloth mills on the Aubette and Robec rivers, subsidiaries of the Seine. New families, such as the Pigache, Mustel and Naguet lineages, rose to prominence among the burgess elite in the thirteenth century.[68]

Rouen emerged as one of the leading cities of north-western Europe in the twelfth and thirteenth centuries, reflecting its commercial importance, its status as a political and religious centre, and the strong municipal organisation provided by the commune. In the mid-fifteenth century, it remained one of the largest cities in France and a melting-pot of people arriving by sea and land, as Charles VII (1422–61) acknowledged in his 1453 statute for Rouen's surgeons.[69] Nonetheless, in the fourteenth and fifteenth centuries a number of crises occurred that affected the city's prosperity and the well-being of its population. In 1346, in the early stages of the Hundred Years' War, Philip VI of France (1328–50) instructed that new walls and ditches should be built to fortify Rouen.[70] Although the direct military impact of the war was not felt until the fifteenth century, the trading activities of Rouen's merchants were disrupted, there was increased taxation, and resources were further stretched due to the influx of dislocated people from the surrounding countryside and destroyed towns such as Pont-de-l'Arche.[71] In October 1359 the future Charles V (1364–80), then duke of Normandy, took steps to assist La Madeleine hospital by exempting it from taxes (octrois), specifically because of the losses sustained (to the hospital's rural possessions) through the destruction wrought by the English. His grant observed that, at the same time, 'the good people of the countryside' were taking refuge there in growing numbers, including the sick and women made pregnant by the enemy.[72]

---

[67] Cartulaire normand de Philippe-Auguste, Louis VIII, Saint-Louis et Philippe-le-Hardi, ed. Léopold Delisle, Caen 1852, repr. Geneva 1978, 26 (no. 154); Sadourny, 'L'Époque', 77.

[68] Sadourny, 'L'Époque', 84–5.

[69] François Hue, La Communauté des chirurgiens de Rouen: chirurgiens – barbiers-chirurgiens – Collège de Chirurgie, 1407–1791, Rouen 1913, 27.

[70] Alain Sadourny, 'Des Débuts de la guerre de cent ans à la Harelle', in Mollat, Histoire de Rouen, 100–1; Gauthiez, 'Urban development', 57.

[71] Sadourny, 'Débuts', 101–2, 118.

[72] 'des bonnes gens du pais': Documents concernant les pauvres de Rouen: extraits des archives de l'hôtel-de-ville, ed. Gustave Panel, Rouen 1917–19, i, pp. xxviii, 3.

Refugees continued to enter Rouen as the Hundred Years' War progressed, particularly following the fall of Harfleur in 1415 and during the English siege of Rouen from July 1418 to January 1419. The siege marked a period of particular hardship, since Henry V of England (1413–22) achieved success by starving the city's inhabitants.[73] As in so many other parts of Europe, the population of early fifteenth-century Rouen was already depleted as a result of the Black Death and subsequent plague epidemics.[74] According to the *Normanniae nova chronica* (surveying the period 473 to 1378), after the plague's arrival in the city in June 1348, between late August and Christmas of that year more than 100,000 people died.[75] Many further plague outbreaks occurred between 1362 and 1523.[76] The chronicle of Pierre Cochon (ending in 1430) claims that new cemeteries were built to serve the parishes of Saint-Vivien and Saint-Maclou at the time of the first epidemic of 1348; the cemetery of Saint-Maclou, a heavily populated parish, was subsequently enlarged repeatedly up to the 1520s.[77] From 1526, with building work completed between 1529 and 1533, wooden galleries were built to serve as a charnel house, which still stands today. The galleries are famous for their carvings of macabre subjects such as the dance of death, skulls, bones and gravediggers' spades.[78]

In addition to feeling the effects of war and pestilence, in the later Middle Ages the people of Rouen suffered as a result of popular uprisings provoked by heavy taxation (culminating in the Harelle revolt of February 1382), flooding (in 1373 and 1382) and severe winters (1362–3 and 1407).[79] In a period in which there was also increasing anxiety about the transmission of disease, and growing hostility towards the vagrant poor, the leprous and other categories of the sick and destitute became less of a focus of Christian charity during this period. Nonetheless, while acknowledging that the generosity that had been exhibited towards lepers in the thirteenth century did not

---

[73] Anne Curry, 'Les Villes normandes et l'occupation anglaise: l'importance du siège de Rouen (1418–1419)', in Bouet and Neveux, *Les Villes normandes*, 112, 114–16. On refugees flocking to Rouen in the 1410s and 1420s see also Lucien René Delsalle, *Rouen et les Rouennais au temps de Jeanne d'Arc, 1400–1470*, Rouen 1982, 71.

[74] Anne Curry suggests that, at the time of Henry V's siege, Rouen had a population of at least 20,000, in contrast to between 40,000 and 70,000 inhabitants in the mid-thirteenth century: *Les Villes normandes*, 111–12.

[75] *Normanniae nova chronica*, 33.

[76] Jean Fournée, 'Les Normands face à la peste', *Le Pays bas-normand* cxlix (1978), 35, 36; Sadourny, 'Débuts', 100; Louis Porquet, *La Peste en normandie du XIVe au XVIIe siècle*, Vire 1898, 124, 128.

[77] *Chronique normande de Pierre Cochon, notaire apostolique à Rouen*, ed. Charles de Robillard de Beaurepaire, Rouen 1870, 73–4.

[78] Nicétas Periaux, *Dictionnaire indicateur et historique des rues et places de Rouen*, Rouen 1870, 574; Sabine Delanes, 'L'Aître Saint-Maclou', in Christiane Decaëns, Henry Decaëns, Jérôme Decoux and Sabine Delanes, *L'Église et l'aître Saint-Maclou, Rouen, Haute-Normandie*, [Rouen] 2012, 56–9, 62–71.

[79] Sadourny, 'Débuts', 100, 118–21.

persist on the same scale in the next two hundred years, this book considers how and why this group was still receiving support as late as the end of the sixteenth century.

This book consists of five chapters that focus particularly on the principal institutions that provided for lepers in medieval Rouen, Mont-aux-Malades and Salle-aux-Puelles. Appendices provide a note on sources and a list of charters and other documents relating to leprosy in Rouen between the twelfth and fifteenth centuries, many of which are as yet unedited. The situation at Rouen is frequently compared to provision for lepers in other major cities of medieval Western Europe, and is placed in the context of the scholarship on leprosy, charity and Normandy. The first chapter surveys the origins and early development of Mont-aux-Malades, the leper house to which the vast majority of the documents relate. This was one of the most distinguished and wealthy *leprosaria* in medieval France, patronised by the Anglo-Norman royal family and aristocracy in the twelfth century. Chapter 2 focuses on the next hundred years, when Mont-aux-Malades received numerous donations from Rouen's burgesses, and after 1204 was also supported by the French kings. By the end of the thirteenth century, the leper house had amassed substantial possessions both within the city of Rouen and in Upper Normandy. This chapter also describes the resident community, composed of not only male and female lepers, but also Augustinian canons and lay brothers and sisters, as well the itinerant lepers that the house was sheltering by the late fourteenth century.

Chapter 3 examines the other communities of lepers around Rouen, especially the female house of Salle-aux-Puelles. These leper houses were much smaller than Mont-aux-Malades, and in some cases had only a brief existence. Although many fewer documentary sources survive for Salle-aux-Puelles than for Mont-aux-Malades, the *Register* of Eudes Rigaud (the record of this archbishop's visitations) provides rich information about this community in the mid-thirteenth century. While Salle-aux-Puelles was the only *leprosarium* solely for women in Normandy, a handful of female leper houses existed in England, providing a broader context for our understanding of this institution.

Chapter 4 addresses the medical world of medieval Rouen, and charts changing responses to leprosy between the twelfth and fifteenth centuries. Medical practitioners were present in the city as early as the tenth century, and by the thirteenth century physicians and surgeons practised there. In terms of medical treatment for leprosy, palliative care was provided in *leprosaria* through dietary regulation, exercise, the provision of clothing and shelter, and sometimes bloodletting. As in other European cities, the diagnosis of suspected cases of leprosy was an increasingly important duty of physicians and surgeons from the thirteenth century. In the fourteenth century, especially following the Black Death, leprosy featured in concerns about the transmission of disease and the public health of the city.

The final chapter examines the religious dimensions of life in Rouen's leper houses, in terms of liturgical practice and the use of sacred space, and the care of the souls of lepers, non-leprous residents and benefactors. Bodily care and spiritual care were closely interlinked, and it was considered particularly important to provide for the souls of lepers, who pursued a religious vocation within the leper house. This chapter highlights the importance of Mont-aux-Malades as a site of burial and commemoration, and the manner in which multiple forms of piety were enacted at Rouen's *leprosaria*. It demonstrates how responses to leprosy were deeply embedded within the religious culture of central and late medieval Rouen.

Overall, the chapters that follow explore both the juncture between leprosy and charity, at a time when assisting lepers was very fashionable, and the broader complexity of attitudes to lepers. Indeed, leprosy sufferers were feared and marginalised in these centuries as well as being an object of philanthropy. The history of Rouen's leper houses and leper communities thus sheds light on the complex relationships between individuals, groups and institutions that shaped society in this period.

1

Rouen's Principal Leper House: Mont-aux-Malades and its Endowment

Although many of the institutions that provided for lepers in the Middle Ages have left little trace in the historical record, Rouen's most prominent *leprosarium*, Mont-aux-Malades, is known to us through its rich archive and architectural remains. The archive sheds light on not only the possessions and activities of the *leprosarium*, but also the charitable practices of Rouen's urban and ecclesiastical elites, particularly in the twelfth and thirteenth centuries. It complements the archives of Rouen's other religious institutions in this period, all of which reveal the social networks, religious culture and patterns of property tenure that shaped life in the medieval city.[1]

Mont-aux-Malades was probably established in the first third of the twelfth century; it stood on a hill north-west of Rouen, in the area now known as Mont-Saint-Aignan. The church of Saint-Thomas, which served the leper community from the later twelfth century, is a functioning parish church today, while the nave of the earlier twelfth-century church of Saint-Jacques is also still standing. As seen elsewhere, such as the site of the leper house of St Nicholas at Harbledown, outside Canterbury, where today there are almshouses for the elderly, the Rouen site still has a welfare function: the maternity hospital *Le Bellevedère* is adjacent to the church of Saint-Thomas.

Mont-aux-Malades could well have originated as a group of lepers living together on a piece of available land, as did the *leprosarium* at Évreux, where the community gradually became institutionalised over the course of the twelfth century.[2] By the mid-twelfth century, Mont-aux-Malades was organised as an Augustinian priory dedicated to St James. The *leprosarium*'s subsequent development was due to the support of high-status lay and ecclesiastical patrons, above all that of members of the Anglo-Norman royal family. From the late twelfth century, following the rededication of Mont-aux-Malades to St Thomas Becket by Henry II (king of England [1154–89] and duke of

---

[1]   See, for example, ADSM, 14H (archive of the abbey of Saint-Ouen, Rouen), 26HP (archive of the priory of Saint-Lô, Rouen), 27HP (archive of the abbey of La Trinité-du-Mont, Rouen), 55H (archive of the abbey of Saint-Amand, Rouen). For recent analyses of material from these archives see various papers in Hicks and Brenner, *Society and culture*, especially those by Grégory Combalbert and Manon Six.

[2]   Tabuteau, 'Une Léproserie normande', 62, 76, 97, 99–100, and 'Histoire et archéologie de la lèpre et des lépreux en Europe et en Méditerranée du moyen âge au temps modernes: 2e table ronde du Groupe de Göttingen', AN xlix (1999), 572.

Normandy [1150–89]) in about 1174, Mont-aux-Malades became a focus of the charity of Rouen's burgess elite, a group that was becoming increasingly well-established and powerful at this time. The burgesses' gifts made the *leprosarium* community a significant property-owner within the city of Rouen, and thus linked it to the commercial and political activities of urban society.

Origins and early history

As for the vast majority of *leprosaria*, there is no extant founding deed for Mont-aux-Malades. The earliest documentary reference to Rouen's lepers is a charter of Geoffrey of Anjou, issued as duke of Normandy (1144–50), reconfirming the grant by Henry I (king of England [1100–35] and duke of Normandy [1106–35]) of 40 *sous* a month to 'the lepers of Rouen'.[3] Although this act does not specifically refer to Mont-aux-Malades, it indicates that, by about 1106–35, a community of lepers at Rouen enjoyed royal patronage. Given the subsequent royal support for Mont-aux-Malades, it appears likely that 'lepers of Rouen' and the leper house were synonymous. Henry I's endowment and his son-in-law's confirmation mark the beginning of the Anglo-Norman royal family's involvement with the city's lepers.

It is possible that, by the late eleventh century or even earlier, lepers had gathered together on this hill outside the walls of Rouen. Leper communities were certainly established in England before 1100: the *leprosarium* at Harbledown was founded by Archbishop Lanfranc of Canterbury (1070–89) in the 1080s, while recent excavations on the site of the leper house of St Mary Magdalen outside Winchester suggest that this may have been an eleventh-century foundation, which could possibly have accommodated lepers before the Norman Conquest.[4] An Augustinian community was established at Mont-aux-Malades in the course of the twelfth century, reflecting the growth of the Augustinian movement, particularly associated with hospitals and leper houses, at this time.[5] The vast majority of medieval *leprosaria* were

---

[3] 'leprosis Rothomagi': appendix 2, no. 21(a).

[4] Edward J. Kealey, *Medieval medicus: a social history of Anglo-Norman medicine*, Baltimore 1981, 85, 86–7. Simon Roffey's archaeological work at Winchester has revealed timber structures underneath twelfth-century masonry buildings on the site of the *leprosarium* of St Mary Magdalen, and a cemetery that also predates the twelfth-century structures. Most of the burials within the cemetery show signs of leprosy; carbon 14 dating indicates that one of these dates from 890–1040, probably 970–1030: 'Medieval leper hospitals', 210–11.

[5] On the influence of the Augustinians in Normandy see Arnoux, 'Les Origines'.

located outside urban settlements.[6] Although this pattern accords with the biblical instruction that lepers should live 'without the camp', there were many other, more practical, reasons for the topography of *leprosaria*. Land outside the city was cheaper and more readily available. A community of lepers required agricultural land to sustain itself, and a reliable water supply. Leper hospitals in semi-rural locations were also able to attract gifts of alms from passing travellers. Mont-aux-Malades, like so many similar institutions, was located close to a major road, that which connected Dieppe and Rouen, an advantage which also facilitated contact with the city.[7]

The siting of Mont-aux-Malades on a hill is also significant. Other *leprosaria* and monastic houses had hilltop locations, such as the leper houses of Bartlemas, outside Oxford, St Nicholas at Harbledown, and Saint-Thomas at Aizier, and the abbey of La-Trinité-du-Mont at Rouen. Such a location increased the visibility of the institution within the landscape, and may also reflect ideas about the salutary benefits of good air.[8] In medieval medicine, the quality of the environment, including the air, was among Galen's non-naturals, external phenomena and psychological states which were understood to cause or prevent disease.[9] Given the increasing concern in the later Middle Ages about the role of corrupt (miasmatic) air in spreading disease, it is likely that therapeutic value was already attributed to pure air by the twelfth century or earlier. The account of Archbishop Eudes Rigaud's visit to the abbey of Bec-Hellouin on 3 April 1268, when arrangements were made for a monk suspected of having leprosy to be sent to a dependent priory, a place 'where there is not the crowding of people, and where he can have the benefit of the air and much mitigation of his infirmity', certainly indicates beliefs about the health-giving importance of good air.[10] The lepers of Mont-aux-Malades lived in an unpolluted and tranquil setting, features which may well have been seen as beneficial to their palliative care. The *leprosarium*'s location may thus reflect ideas about how the leprous could best be cared for, as well as cohering with the biblical injunction that they should be physically separated.

---

[6] Some *leprosaria* were situated immediately outside city gates, to accommodate lepers who attempted to enter or had been required to leave. At Nuremberg, by 1446, there was a leper hospital within the walls, which sheltered the very sick during the annual *Schau* (examination of vagrant lepers) in Holy Week: Demaitre, *Leprosy*, 45–6.

[7] On the topography of *leprosaria* see Touati, 'La Géographie hospitalière médiévale', 7–20.

[8] Kealey, *Medieval medicus*, 85, 86–7.

[9] Faith Wallis (ed.), *Medieval medicine: a reader*, Toronto 2010, 485–6, 548; Christopher A. Bonfield, 'The *Regimen sanitatis* and its dissemination in England, c. 1348–1550', unpubl. PhD diss. East Anglia 2006, 1–6.

[10] 'ubi non est frequentia hominum, ubique beneficium aeris et multa infirmitatis sue levimenta habere posset': *Regestrum*, 623; *Register*, 717.

The only extensive account to date of the history of Mont-aux-Malades, published in 1851, was written by Pierre Langlois, a priest who taught at the seminary located at Mont-aux-Malades in the nineteenth century.[11] Langlois followed the view of earlier historians of Rouen, such as François Farin and Antoine-Nicolas Servin, that the *leprosarium* was established by a group of urban parishes in 1131, which exclusively held the right to send leprous parishioners there. These were apparently known as the *paroisses du Droit*.[12] Farin lists twenty parish churches (a further church is added by Langlois) which, he claims, financed the foundation of Mont-aux-Malades and endowed it with a fief in the area south-east of Rouen that spanned Sotteville-sous-le-Val (near Pont de l'Arche), Les Authieux, Pîtres and Yonville.[13]

Almost all these parishes were located within Rouen's late twelfth-century walls.[14] Rouen had thirty-two parishes in total at this time (prior to the suppression of that of Saint-Clément by Eudes Rigaud in 1251), meaning that a majority of the parishes, two-thirds, would have had this connection to Mont-aux-Malades.[15] The city's four oldest parishes (Saint-Herbland,

---

[11] Pierre Langlois, *Histoire du prieuré du Mont-aux-Malades-lès-Rouen, et correspondance du prieur de ce monastère avec saint Thomas de Cantorbéry, 1120–1820*, Rouen 1851; Philippe Deschamps, 'L'Abbé Cochet, l'abbé Langlois et la formation archéologique du clergé diocésain au XIXe siècle', in *Centenaire de l'abbé Cochet 1975: actes du colloque international d'archéologie, Rouen 3–4–5 juillet 1975*, Rouen 1978, i. 29. See also Philippe Deschamps, 'Léproseries et maladreries rouennaises: le prieuré du Mont-aux-Malades et ses rapports avec Thomas Becket', *Revue des Sociétés Savantes de Haute-Normandie* xlviii (1967), 31–46.

[12] Langlois, *Histoire*, 2, 118 n. 1; François Farin, *Histoire de la ville de Rouen:divisée en six parties*, 3rd edn, Rouen 1731, ii/5, p. 40; ii/6, p. 26; Antoine-Nicolas Servin, *Histoire de la ville de Rouen, capitale du pays et duché de Normandie, depuis sa fondation jusqu'en l'année 1774: suivie d'un essai sur la Normandie littéraire*, Rouen 1775, i. 12.

[13] The twenty parishes were Notre-Dame-de-la-Ronde, Saint-Amand, Saint-André-aux-Fèvres, Saint-Cande-le-Jeune, Sainte-Croix-Saint-Ouen, Saint-Éloi, Saint-Étienne-la-Grande-Église, Saint-Étienne-des-Tonneliers, Saint-Herbland, Saint-Lô, Saint-Martin-du-Pont, Saint-Martin-sur-Renelle, Saint-Michel, Saint-Nicolas, Saint-Patrice, Saint-Pierre-du-Châtel, Saint-Pierre-le-Portier, Saint-Sauveur, Saint-Vigor, Saint-Vincent: Farin, *Histoire*, ii/6, p. 26. Langlois (*Histoire*, 118 n. 1) adds the parish of Saint-Jean[-sur-Renelle]. See Bruno Tabuteau, 'Combien de lépreux au moyen âge? Essai d'étude quantitative appliquée à la lèpre: les exemples de Rouen et de Bellencombre au XIIIe siècle', *Sources: Travaux Historiques* xiii (1988), 22 n. 7. Tabuteau states that the parish of Saint-Jean is mentioned in an *acte du tabellionage de Rouen* of 3 February 1478 in ADSM.

[14] In about 1131 Sainte-Croix-Saint-Ouen and Saint-Vigor were located just outside the city walls, while Saint-Pierre-le-Portier was situated on the western city wall: Gauthiez, 'Paris, un Rouen capétien?', 119; Bates, 'Rouen', 2; Servin, *Histoire*, i. 8, 10.

[15] Vincent Tabbagh, 'L'Exercise de la fonction curiale à Rouen au XVe siècle', in Éric Barré (ed.), *La Paroisse en Normandie au moyen âge: la vie paroissiale, l'église et le cimetière: histoire, art, archéologie*, Saint-Lô 2008, 48 and n. 5. Tabbagh refers to parishes within the city walls; according to Lemoine and Tanguy there were thirty-six parishes at the end of the Middle Ages: *Rouen*, p. 12.

Notre-Dame-de-la-Ronde, Saint-Étienne-la-grande-Église and Saint-Lô), and parishes in the affluent area of the *Vieux Marché* (Saint-Michel, Saint-Sauveur, Saint-Éloi, Saint-André-aux-Fèvres and Saint-Vincent) were among the *paroisses du Droit*, indicating that the inhabitants of the most ancient, wealthy parts of the city could have been particularly responsible for this initiative.[16] In general, too, most of the twenty-one parishes were located in the northern and western parts of the city, areas in which Mont-aux-Malades increasingly acquired property in the thirteenth century.

The establishment of urban leper houses elsewhere was attributed to collective civic efforts: Le Popelin at Sens, for example, is understood to have been founded by the burgesses and inhabitants of Sens. According to a document of 1412, the *leprosarium* of Saint-Lazare at Aumône near Pontoise, in existence before 1137, was established by the burgesses of Pontoise.[17] This document marks the entrance of a leprous man, who had the right to be admitted to the hospital for life because he was born in Pontoise.[18] It is traditionally held that the *leprosarium* of St Stephen's, outside Dublin, was founded by the people of Dublin; the mayor and civic government were its patrons from the Anglo-Norman period onwards.[19] Although the leper hospital of Saint-Gilles, Pont-Audemer, was founded by Waleran, count of Meulan, in about 1135, from an early stage the burgesses of Pont-Audemer were involved in selecting those patients who were admitted.[20] Regarding Mont-aux-Malades, however, Langlois acknowledges that 'The date of the transaction between the parishes and the priory is uncertain.'[21] The *paroisses du Droit* are not mentioned in any document until the end of the fourteenth century, in a charter of Charles VI of France (1380–1422) issued on 18 June 1393, which refers to the responsibility of Mont-aux-Malades to welcome and sustain, for as long as they lived, all the lepers from twenty-one parishes of Rouen.[22] At the same time, however, the king describes the *leprosarium* as a royal foun-

---

[16] Servin, *Histoire*, i. 5–6.

[17] Francis Molard, *Inventaire-sommaire des archives départementales antérieures à 1790: Yonne: archives hospitalières – série H supplément*, iv, Auxerre 1897, pp. l–li; agreement issued by Simon Paine, mayor of Pontoise, for the admission of Jehan Duquesnoy called 'le Bourgignon' to the *leprosarium* of Saint-Lazare at Aumône near Pontoise, 17 May 1412, Wellcome Library, London, MS 5133/1; Touati, *Archives de la lèpre*, 320.

[18] Wellcome Library, MS 5133/1.

[19] Myles V. Ronan, 'St Stephen's hospital, Dublin', *Dublin Historical Record* iv (1941–2), 142; Lee, *Leper hospitals in medieval Ireland*, 47.

[20] In about 1150 Waleran of Meulan issued a mandate to the leading citizens of Pont-Audemer, revealing that, in return for delivering the customs due on leather and a weekly tax from every house in the town, the citizens had a say in the admission of lepers to Saint-Gilles: Mesmin, 'Waleran, count of Meulan', 15–16.

[21] 'L'Époque de la transaction entre les paroisses et le prieuré est incertaine': Langlois, *Histoire*, 118 n. 1.

[22] AN, Paris, S4889B, dossier 13, no. 14; Langlois, *Histoire*, 118 n. 1.

dation.[23] This suggests that Mont-aux-Malades's origins were most strongly associated with the endowment of Henry I and the subsequent patronage of the Anglo-Norman royal family; the French kings would have inherited this connection with the leper house when they assumed direct control of Normandy in 1204.[24] Almost certainly, therefore, Mont-aux-Malades was not actually founded by twenty-one Rouen parishes; nonetheless, a special relationship with these parishes was evidently in place by the end of the fourteenth century. It is possible that links with particular parishes were forged in the course of the thirteenth century, as Mont-aux-Malades developed property interests in certain areas of the city. Parishes whose inhabitants were generous to the *leprosarium* might have been accorded special rights to send leprous parishioners there, strengthening the ties between the leper community and the city.

Patronage for Mont-aux-Malades in the twelfth century

Royal patronage
In the twelfth century the Anglo-Norman rulers were actively engaged in charitable patronage, underlining not only their piety and concern for their future salvation, but also their sense of responsibility for the needy, and political skill in publicly demonstrating these attributes. Charity also served a political purpose by reinforcing the bonds between Anglo-Norman nobles and their lords, since lords may in many cases have instructed their vassals to endow particular institutions.[25] Simultaneously, it strengthened family ties within the royal lineage, and family identity by means of commemoration, as fathers, mothers, sons and daughters collaborated in endowing worthy institutions, often in memory of deceased ancestors.[26] Henry I and his successors were certainly not the only monarchs to engage in the practice of charity. Louis VI (1108–37) and Louis VII (1137–80), for example, were major benefactors of the *leprosarium* of Saint-Lazare outside Paris, which may well have been a royal foundation.[27]

Coinciding with the emergence of the first *leprosaria* in Western Europe,

---

[23] AN, Paris, S4889B, dossier 13, no. 14.

[24] For evidence of how the association with having founded a *leprosarium* was transferred from English to French monarchs after 1204 see how in 1366 Charles V of France donated Salle-aux-Puelles, endowed by Henry II in the 1180s, to Rouen's La Madeleine hospital: appendix 2, nos 13(a), 13(b).

[25] On the manner in which the support of aristocrats encouraged their tenants to patronise Rievaulx abbey see Jamroziak, *Rievaulx abbey*, 62.

[26] On royal and aristocratic practices of commemoration see Brenner, Cohen and Franklin-Brown, *Memory and commemoration*, pt IV.

[27] *Recueil d'actes de Saint-Lazare de Paris, 1124–1254*, ed. Simone Lefèvre, under the direction of Lucie Fossier, Paris, pp. x–xi, xvii.

the beneficence of the Anglo-Norman royal family towards lepers appears to have originated with Henry I and his wives, Matilda of Scotland (queen from 1100 to 1118) and Adeliza of Louvain (queen from 1121 to 1135).[28] Queen Matilda, the daughter of St Margaret of Scotland, was reputed to have shown particular charity to the leprous. The chronicler Aelred of Rievaulx recounted the testimony of David, Matilda's younger brother and later king of Scotland (1124–53), that, during the Easter court of 1105, he witnessed the queen in her apartments kissing lepers and washing their feet.[29] The queen also endowed institutions for lepers. She founded the major *leprosarium* of St Giles at Holborn, outside the city of London, endowed and possibly founded the leper house of St James and St Mary Magdalene at Chichester, and may have supported the house for leprous women at Westminster dedicated to St James.[30]

Henry I established institutions for lepers at Oxford, Shrewsbury, Newcastle and Bridgenorth, and also supported leper houses at Colchester, Lincoln, Reading, Canterbury and, interestingly, Chartres in France.[31] His second queen, Adeliza of Louvain, founded the *leprosarium* of St Giles at Wilton, near the abbey where Matilda of Scotland had been educated.[32] The Empress Matilda, the daughter of Henry I and Matilda of Scotland and the wife of Geoffrey of Anjou, also supported lepers. She granted ninety acres of land to the lepers of Argentan (Orne), a gift reconfirmed by Henry II.[33] Following an illness related to the birth of her second son, Geoffrey, at Rouen in May 1134, the empress 'did not even hesitate to dispose of the silk mattress on which she had slept during her illness, but sold it and ordered the money she received to be given to lepers'.[34] The lepers of Rouen, indeed those of

---

[28] Kealey, *Medieval medicus*, 89–95.

[29] Lois L. Huneycutt, *Matilda of Scotland: a study in medieval queenship*, Woodbridge 2003, 104–5; Catherine Peyroux, 'The leper's kiss', in Sharon Farmer and Barbara H. Rosenwein (eds), *Monks and nuns, saints and outcasts: religion in medieval society: essays in honor of Lester K. Little*, Ithaca, NY 2000, 183; Kealey, *Medieval medicus*, 19–20, 90.

[30] Huneycutt, *Matilda of Scotland*, 105–6; Kealey, *Medieval medicus*, 89–91.

[31] For Chartres see *Cartulaire de la léproserie du Grand-Beaulieu et du prieuré de Notre-Dame de la Bourdinière*, ed. René Merlet and Maurice Jusselin, Chartres 1909, 1 (no. 1), 2 (no. 2), 5 (no. 11), 13 (no. 28).

[32] Kealey, *Medieval medicus*, 20–1, 93–5; Huneycutt, *Matilda of Scotland*, 18–21.

[33] For the letters of Henry II confirming his mother's grant to the lepers of Argentan see *The letters and charters of King Henry II (1154–1189)*, ed. Nicholas Vincent and others, Oxford forthcoming, no. 67 (provisional number). The beneficiary of the empress's grant could well have been the leper house of Sainte-Madeleine of Argentan, on which see Jean Fournée, 'Les Maladreries et les vocables de leurs chapelles', *Lèpre et lépreux en Normandie, Cahiers Léopold Delisle* xlvi (1997), 99.

[34] 'nec a culcicra serica, super quam in ipsa infirmitate iacebat, abstineret, quin ipsa distracta pretium eius leprosis erogari iuberet': *The 'Gesta normannorum ducum' of William of Jumièges, Orderic Vitalis, and Robert of Torigni*, ed. and trans. Elisabeth van Houts, Oxford 1992–5, ii. 244–5; *Chronique de Robert de Torigni*, i. 192–3; Marjorie Chibnall, *The Empress Matilda: queen consort, queen mother and lady of the English*, Oxford 1991, 188

Mont-aux-Malades, could well have been the beneficiaries of this gift, which was valuable and symbolic.[35] The mattress must have fetched a large sum of money, since it was a luxury item, associated with the empress and the birth of her son. The link with healing was also significant, since although contemporaries were aware that lepers did not recover from their sickness, *leprosaria* aimed to alleviate physical, as well as spiritual, suffering. There may here be an interesting parallel with the charity of the empress's mother, whose foundation of the leper house of St Giles at Holborn may have been connected to a difficult pregnancy. Indeed, the empress was continuing a tradition of female piety in her family, emulating the charity of her mother and her grandmother, St Margaret of Scotland, who herself established a hospital at Edinburgh, and set an example through almsgiving, fasting, and concern for orphans and prisoners.[36] Both the empress and Matilda of Scotland assumed duties of government, and they might also have viewed their charitable activities as part of their responsibilities towards public order and welfare.[37]

Matilda held her court at Rouen in the latter years of her life until her death in 1167, and was particularly attached to the city. She lived on the other side of the Seine at Quevilly, either in the ducal palace built by Henry I (where Salle-aux-Puelles would be established in the 1180s) or in guest accommodation in the nearby priory of Notre-Dame-du-Pré, a dependency of Bec-Hellouin.[38] The empress heavily financed the construction of the first stone bridge across the Seine at Rouen, an essential civic amenity. Geoffrey of Anjou had previously restored the wooden bridge, and Matilda left money in her will for the completion of a stone bridge, which remained in place until the sixteenth century.[39] In late 1164 Prior Nicholas of Mont-aux-Malades met the empress twice in his capacity as Thomas Becket's envoy, suggesting that she was acquainted with the leper community and its affairs.[40]

The Empress Matilda may well have inspired and encouraged the patronage of other members of the Anglo-Norman royal family, particularly

---

(stating that the mattress was donated in 1161 but the gift appears to be much earlier – dating from soon after May 1134); Langlois, *Histoire*, 12.

[35] According to Marjorie Chibnall 'she gave her silk mattress to be sold for the leper hospital of St James at Rouen [i.e. Mont-aux-Malades]': *Empress Matilda*, 188. However, the description of the event by Robert of Torigni only refers to a gift on behalf of 'lepers'.

[36] Kealey, *Medieval medicus*, 89–90; Chibnall, *Empress Matilda*, 11.

[37] See Chibnall, *Empress Matilda*, 10, 11.

[38] Ibid. 151.

[39] Musset 'Rouen', 56; Bates, 'Rouen', 5; *Chronique de Robert de Torigni*, i. 239, 368; Chibnall, *Empress Matilda*, 152. Here is another parallel with the good works of Matilda of Scotland, who built stone bridges in Essex over the river Lea: Kealey, *Medieval medicus*, 20; Chibnall, *Empress Matilda*, 152 n. 52.

[40] Prior Nicholas to Thomas Becket, Christmas season, 1164, *CTB* i. 158–69 (no. 41) at pp. 162–9; Chibnall, *Empress Matilda*, 169–71.

her son Henry II, for Mont-aux-Malades in the twelfth century. Matilda's youngest son, William, and Henry II's second cousin, Henry de Sully, fifth abbot of Fécamp (1139–88), both supported the leper community. In 1154 Henry de Sully donated four acres of land in the fief of the priory of Saint-Gervais, Rouen, to the lepers of Rouen, at the request of Henry II, Hugh of Amiens, archbishop of Rouen (1130–64), the Empress Matilda and the burgesses of Rouen.[41] Between summer 1158 and his death on 29 January 1164, Prince William donated 40 *sous* annual rent to Mont-aux-Malades from his revenues at Dieppe, for the salvation of himself, his ancestors and his brother Geoffrey (who died on 26 July 1158).[42] The Empress Matilda was the first witness of his act, which suggests that she may have overseen or instigated it.[43] Since Matilda had sold her mattress on behalf of lepers on the occasion of Geoffrey's birth, it presumably made sense for his brother to endow the leper community of Mont-aux-Malades for the sake of Geoffrey's soul after his death. William's grant of 40 *sous* a year echoes his grandfather Henry I's earlier gift of 40 *sous* a month, further indicating that the prince was acting within a family tradition of patronage for Mont-aux-Malades.

Matilda's eldest son, Henry II, was undoubtedly the most prominent twelfth-century patron of Mont-aux-Malades. He issued seven acts in the leper house's favour between 1156 and 1189, instituted its annual eight-day fair (probably in the 1150s), and refounded it in about 1174, in dedication to the recently canonised Thomas Becket.[44] While his support should be seen in the context of his religious patronage more broadly, which benefited the Carthusians, Cistercians, Grandmontines and other orders, as well as a number of hospitals and leper communities in England, Normandy and Anjou, Mont-aux-Malades was one of the institutions to which the king was most generous.[45] Henry II's gifts created estates for Mont-aux-Malades in Upper Normandy, established vital revenues and resources for the leper house, and testify to the king's keen interest in Rouen and his concern for lepers. They also show how he used charity to reinforce his lordship,

---

[41] Appendix 2, no. 33; Langlois, *Histoire*, 12. During Henry de Sully's long abbacy, the *leprosarium* at Aizier (Eure) was established on land belonging to the abbey of Fécamp. The house at Aizier was dedicated to St Thomas Becket, and its chapel was probably built between 1173 and 1180.

[42] Appendix 2, no. 104; Langlois, *Histoire*, 12; W. L. Warren, *Henry II*, London 1973, 76; *Chronique de Robert de Torigni*, i. 350.

[43] Appendix 2, no. 104.

[44] The exact date of Henry II's refoundation of Mont-aux-Malades is not known; given that much of his monastic patronage after Becket's murder dates from the end of the 1170s and beginning of the 1180s, it is possible that the leper house was refounded slightly later than 1174: Elizabeth M. Hallam, 'Henry II as a founder of monasteries', *Journal of Ecclesiastical History* xxviii (1977), 131.

[45] Ibid. 117–29, esp. p. 115 which notes that Henry II only 'occasionally granted lands, pensions and financial help' to monastic houses. Mont-aux-Malades was one of this select group of monasteries.

disposing of his Norman lands and, it would appear, instructing and over-seeing gifts by members of his nobility.

In his earliest charter for Mont-aux-Malades, issued between 1156 and April 1166, Henry confirmed an annual grant of barley from the mill of Longpaon (near Darnétal, east of Rouen) to the lepers by Osbert, lord of Préaux, in return for the lepers' acceptance of Osbert's claim to half the mill, from which they were accustomed to enjoy an annual income.[46] From 1165 onwards the king made direct grants, indicating that, perhaps influenced by his mother, who died on 10 September 1167, he was assuming responsibility for the royal family's patronage of the *leprosarium*.[47] Henry granted several possessions in the fertile Pays de Caux, in Upper Normandy, establishing significant landed interests for Mont-aux-Malades in this area. Between February 1165 and 1173, the king donated a piece of land in the forest of Lillebonne, near Bolbec.[48] In the same period, possibly before March 1170, he granted the church of Saint-Sauveur at Nointot (in the west of the Pays de Caux), at the request of John de Mara and his wife, patrons of the church, who had placed it in Henry's hands at the beseeching of his eldest son Henry (who was crowned the Young King on 14 June 1170).[49] In the same act, Henry II confirmed to Mont-aux-Malades land at Bolleville (near Nointot), donated by its lord, R. de Thieouville, and land at Drosay (in the *département* of Manche), held by Richard de Osqueville.[50]

Between 1170 and 1173 Henry II donated the church of Saint-Martin at Beuzeville-la-Grenier to Mont-aux-Malades, thus conferring another posses-sion in the immediate vicinity of Nointot.[51] Simultaneously, he granted land in the parish of Saint-Martin de Beuzeville-la-Grenier which Hugh, his steward, had held from him, who had restored it to Henry 'so that I might give it to them [God and the brothers of Mont-aux-Malades]'.[52] This language closely resembles that of Henry II's act donating the church of Saint-Sauveur at Nointot ('they [the church's patrons] placed it in my hands ... so that I might give it to the said brothers'), indicating the symbolic importance of a gift being made through the mediation of the king, as well as suggesting that the king had instructed both gifts.[53]

After his coronation, the Young King issued his own charter confirming

---

[46] Appendix 2, no. 30(a).

[47] 'The empress lived until 1167 ... exercising until the end a strong influence on her son [Henry II]': Warren, *Henry II*, 81.

[48] Appendix 2, no. 30(c).

[49] Ibid. no. 30(b).

[50] Ibid.

[51] Ibid. no. 30(d).

[52] 'ut eam eis darem': ibid.

[53] 'qui eam in manu mea posuerunt ... ut eam darem predictis fratribus': appendix 2, no. 30(b), transcribed from *Letters and charters of King Henry II*, no. 2280 (provisional number).

that John de Mara had granted the church at Nointot at his request.[54] This evidences how charitable donations could result from networks of patronage implicating several members of the Anglo-Norman royal family and nobility. Even though the Young King twice rebelled against his father, many of his charters repeated or confirmed provisions of Henry II, and this appears to be the case with regard to the gift to Mont-aux-Malades.[55] Henry the Young King also supported Rouen's La Madeleine hospital, taking it under his protection. After his death on 11 June 1183, men loyal to him, including Gerard Talbot and Henry, count of Eu, made gifts to La Madeleine for the sake of the Young King's soul. It has been argued that Henry II imposed these gifts on the Young King's men as punishment for their support of his son's 1183 revolt.[56] This interesting interpretation suggests that the royal imposition of charitable gifts could reflect forcible coercion and could play a part in the re-assertion of royal authority following political upheaval.

One of the most significant of Henry II's charters for Mont-aux-Malades, of which the original and numerous later copies survive, was issued between May 1172 and July 1178, possibly before May 1175. It confirms the leper community's right to hold an annual fair from 1 to 8 September and grants a rent of 60 *livres*, 6 *sous*, 8 *deniers* and 3,000 herrings from the *vicomté* of Rouen, 140 acres of land in the forest of Lyons and further lands in the Pays de Caux.[57] These were substantial gifts, indicating the king's heightened interest in Mont-aux-Malades following the martyrdom of Thomas Becket (29 December 1170) and his canonisation (21 February 1173). Becket had been a close friend of Prior Nicholas of Mont-aux-Malades, and the community prayed on his behalf in the first months of his exile from England.[58] Henry II's generous patronage for Mont-aux-Malades after December 1170 must be understood in the context of this link with Becket and the king's penance for the archbishop's murder, as well as his family's longstanding interest in Rouen's lepers.

Although Henry II had inaugurated Mont-aux-Malades' fair at an earlier date, probably between 1151 and 1154, in this document he specified the particular benefits which were to accrue to the leper house, and to himself,

---

[54] Appendix 2, no. 31.

[55] R. J. Smith, 'Henry II's heir: the *acta* and seal of Henry the Young King, 1170–83', *English Historical Review* cxvi (2001), 297–8.

[56] Rousseau, 'L'Assistance charitable', i. 6–8. The Young King's charter for La Madeleine hospital is not cited in R. J. Smith's list of the Young King's *acta*, and its date is unclear: according to Rousseau, it survives only as a copy in a manuscript history of La Madeleine. Smith confirms that Gerard Talbot was among 'the Young Henry's long-term supporters and household men': 'Henry II's heir', 300.

[57] Appendix 2, no. 30(e).

[58] Nicholas to Becket, Christmas season, 1164, CTB i. 158–69 (no. 41) at pp. 160–1; Langlois, *Histoire*, 20.

during this event.[59] The profits from the fair were to be divided equally between the king and the lepers. While the fair was in session, half the customs on all products entering Rouen, by land or water, were to be enjoyed by the lepers and half by the king. The customs at the fair were to be set at the same rate as the current customs of Rouen.[60] It is noteworthy that the king established his own financial interest in the fair: this demonstrates how the proffering of charity could be carefully calculated, to result in material as well as spiritual benefits for the benefactor.

The rededication of Mont-aux-Malades

The king's greatest act of patronage was his refoundation of the *leprosarium* in dedication to Becket, when he built a new church and more extensive claustral buildings for the community.[61] The new complex incorporated the parish church of Saint-Gilles, established between 1154 and 1165 for the poor living around the leper house, which was now used for the burial of leprous canons.[62] In turn, the original priory church of Saint-Jacques assumed parochial functions at Mont-aux-Malades.[63]

This act occurred after Henry II's visit to Becket's tomb at Canterbury on 12 July 1174 and subsequent military victory at Rouen on 14 August, when he defeated a rebellion led by the Young King Henry, Eleanor of Aquitaine and Louis VII.[64] The refoundation might well have been specifically motivated by Mont-aux-Malades' location at Rouen, the city over which Henry regained control after apparently seeking the new saint's intercession at his tomb. At the same time, however, it is possible that Mont-aux-Malades was among the monastic foundations that the king endowed in return for the commutation of the penance that he was required to fulfil by Pope Alexander III at Avranches in 1172. In light of this possibility, it is interesting that Alexander III issued a bull for Mont-aux-Malades following the rededication, confirming the community's possession of the church at Nointot and a mill at Maromme.[65]

Mont-aux-Malades' refoundation also reflects the widespread cult of Thomas Becket which developed immediately following his death, spreading from Canterbury as far as northern Italy.[66] Between 1173 and the end of the

---

[59] Langlois, *Histoire*, 7–8.

[60] Appendix 2, no. 30(e).

[61] Langlois, *Histoire*, 82–4.

[62] Appendix 2, no. 95; Langlois, *Histoire*, 6, 84.

[63] Langlois, *Histoire*, 84–5.

[64] Ibid. 82–4; Warren, *Henry II*, 117–36; Frank Barlow, *Thomas Becket*, London 1986, repr. London 2000, 269–70.

[65] Appendix 2, no. 4.

fourteenth century, fifty-nine churches were dedicated to St Thomas in the ecclesiastical province of Rouen, the majority of these dating from between 1173 and 1220. Thus, Henry's new foundation at Mont-aux-Malades formed part of, and perhaps encouraged, a particularly strong cult of Becket in Normandy, focused above all in the archdiocese of Rouen itself, where twenty-nine of the fifty-nine dedications were located.[67] The king was also involved in the establishment of an Augustinian priory dedicated to Becket at Dublin, and may have refounded hospitals at Argentan and Caen in dedication to the martyr.[68]

After refounding Mont-aux-Malades, Henry took the community under his protection, pledging to protect the church of Saint-Thomas, the lepers, their revenues and possessions, and instructing his men, both ecclesiastical and secular, to do the same.[69] He continued to support the leper house in the latter years of his reign, making an annual grant of 6,000 herrings from the *prévôté* of Dieppe between June 1177 and July 1188.[70] Given that Henry II perpetuated a tradition of family patronage for Rouen's chief leper house, it is striking that his sons, Richard I (1189–99) and John, were much less forthcoming with their support. While Richard issued one charter for Salle-aux-Puelles, no acts by him for Mont-aux-Malades survive.[71] John made no donations, but did reconfirm Henry II's grant of protection on 16 October 1200.[72] Richard's lack of involvement could be explained by the fact that (as in England) he spent little time in Normandy during his peripatetic reign; from 1204 John was no longer duke of Normandy, and was thus no longer connected to Rouen as its lord.

Aristocratic and ecclesiastical patronage

Both during and after Henry II's reign, however, Rouen's lepers received the support of the Anglo-Norman nobility, as well as that of the secular clergy. Henry II's chamberlain, Roscelin, son of Clarembaud, founded a parish church dedicated to St Giles at Mont-aux-Malades between 1154 and 1165, endowed it with 7 *livres* of rent, and arranged for one of the leper house's canons to serve in it.[73] Langlois suggests that this church was needed to serve

---

[66] Langlois, *Histoire*, 85–6.

[67] Raymonde Foreville, 'Les Origines normandes de la famille Becket et le culte de saint Thomas en Normandie', *Mélanges offerts à Pierre Andrieu-Guitrancourt, L'Année Canonique* xvii (1973), 448–9, 452.

[68] Hallam, 'Henry II', 125, 127–8.

[69] Appendix 2, no. 30(f); Langlois, *Histoire*, 84.

[70] Appendix 2, no. 30(g).

[71] Ibid. no. 83.

[72] Ibid. no. 42; Langlois, *Histoire*, 89–90.

[73] Appendix 2, no. 95; Langlois, *Histoire*, 6. The church of Saint-Gilles fell into ruin in the late seventeenth century; there are no architectural remains still standing today.

a community of poor people that had become established around the *lepro-sarium*.[74] At least three members of the Talbot family, an important Anglo-Norman lineage, supported the leper house in the twelfth century.[75] In an undated act, probably issued in 1166, Richard Talbot granted the sale of a house to Mont-aux-Malades in the forecourt of Rouen cathedral by William and Vincent, the sons of Richard, son of Gosbert, and their sister Emma, for 330 marks of silver.[76] This could well be the purchase to which Prior Nicholas referred in his August 1167 letter to Thomas Becket, complaining of the need to enter Rouen almost daily to defer repayment of a debt for a house that he had bought the previous year.[77]

This Richard was surely synonymous with the Richard Talbot to whom Henry II donated land in Herefordshire (1156–April 1157) 'in return for his service', and the clerk of the same name who witnessed the king's charter granting the church of Saint-Sauveur at Nointot to Mont-aux-Malades.[78] The former charter demonstrates that Richard was a faithful vassal of Henry II; the latter charter was issued at Rouen, revealing that he was active in the city. In his authorisation of Mont-aux-Malades' purchase of the house, Richard also relinquished his own right of access to the property. However, he reserved a personal right to receive hospitality there (indicating that rights of hospitality in the ecclesiastical centre of Rouen were much valued). Furthermore, he mentioned an earlier donation of 5 *sous* (annual rent) to the lepers by his father. Like the manner in which the grant of Osbert de Préaux refers to the leper community's earlier rights from the mill of Longpaon, this suggests that the community's endowment began to be formed prior to these documents of the 1150s and 1160s – perhaps in the first third of the twelfth century. It also implies that the Talbot family were among the earliest patrons of Mont-aux-Malades. Richard's sons, Hugh and William, consented to these provisions, while Ralph Talbot was among the witnesses.[79]

A female member of the Talbot family, Cecily, was also a patron of Mont-aux-Malades. In the early 1170s, Gilbert Foliot, bishop of London (1163–87) granted the church of Vange (Essex, diocese of London) to Mont-aux-Malades, on behalf of Lady Cecily Talbot, in whose patrimony the church

[74] Langlois, *Histoire*, 6.

[75] Power, *The Norman frontier*, 295, 504. See p. 29 above for the support of Gerard Talbot, a follower of the Young King Henry, for La Madeleine hospital at Rouen.

[76] Appendix 2, no. 87.

[77] Nicholas to Becket, August 1167, CTB, i. 622–3 (no. 132).

[78] 'pro seruicio suo': Henry II's donation to Richard Talbot, undated [1156–April 1157], *Letters and charters of King Henry II*, no. 2577 (provisional number); appendix 2, no. 30(b); Judith A. Everard, 'Talbot family' (unpublished notes, November 2005). I thank Dr Everard for providing me with information and references regarding the Talbot family.

[79] Appendix 2, no. 87.

was situated.[80] He established the authority of Herbert, prior of Mont-aux-Malades, over the church of Vange, and attached his own seal, that of Cecily Talbot and that of 'St Thomas, a short time previously archbishop of Canterbury' to the charter.[81] This gift was made after Becket's canonisation, but before Mont-aux-Malades' refoundation, since it was conferred on the church of Saint-Jacques and the community. It was a substantial donation – almost all other churches received by Mont-aux-Malades in the twelfth and thirteenth centuries were royal donations – and granted the *leprosarium* its only known possession in England.

This patron was almost certainly Cecily Talbot, dowager countess of Hereford (d. 1207), daughter of Pain fitzJohn and niece and heiress of Geoffrey Talbot II (d. 1140).[82] A confirmation by Henry II of lands in Essex to Maurice fitz Geoffrey of Tilty, issued between 1155 and April 1179, refers to a charter of Cecily Talbot and her second husband, William of Poitou, concerning land in Essex.[83] This confirms Cecily's property interests in this county. While, as bishop of London, it was appropriate for Gilbert Foliot to confirm this transaction, he and Cecily may have been personally acquainted. Gilbert had served as bishop of Hereford between 1148 and 1163; Cecily was married to her first husband, Roger, earl of Hereford, between 1138 and 1155.[84] The bishop's involvement, and his attaching of the seal of St Thomas to the charter, are significant, since he had earlier been one of Becket's leading opponents.[85] This donation thus testifies to Mont-aux-Malades' significance in the Becket cult at an early date, and reflects the social ties among members of the Anglo-Norman elite, in Normandy and England, that lay behind much of the *leprosarium*'s early endowment.

Following the rededication of Mont-aux-Malades, several other members of the Anglo-Norman nobility offered gifts. In the last quarter of the twelfth century, John de Hodenc donated land, with the rent that it returned, at Saint-Gervais, Rouen, to three religious houses: Mont-aux-Malades, Rouen's La Madeleine hospital, and the abbey of Sainte-Marie at Beaubec (in the

---

[80] The church at Vange still stands, and is dedicated to All Saints: Nikolaus Pevsner, rev. Enid Radcliffe, *The buildings of England: Essex*, Harmondsworth 1965, 75. Pevsner mentions the remains of a Norman window and a twelfth- or thirteenth-century font.

[81] 'sancti Thome dudum Cant(uariensis) archiepiscopi': appendix 2, no. 12; *The letters and charters of Gilbert Foliot, abbot of Gloucester (1139–48), bishop of Hereford (1148–63) and London (1163–87)*, ed. Adrian Morey and C. N. L. Brooke, Cambridge 1967, 472 (no. 436).

[82] Ian J. Sanders, *English baronies: a study of their origin and descent, 1086–1327*, Oxford 1960, 144; Power, *The Norman frontier*, 508 n. 5.

[83] Act of Henry II in favour of Maurice fitz Geoffrey of Tilty, n.d. (1155–April 1179/? 1155–September 1176), *Letters and charters of King Henry II*, no. 2651 (provisional number).

[84] Sanders, *English baronies*, 144.

[85] Langlois, *Histoire*, 80.

Pays de Bray, south-east of Dieppe). The three houses were to come into possession of the land and revenue upon the death of John or his wife, Alix.[86] In another charter issued after the leper house's refoundation, Alix, the daughter of Osbert de Préaux and widow of John de Hodenc, confirmed this donation following her husband's death.[87] The de Préaux, like the Talbots, were a distinguished Anglo-Norman family – we have already seen that Osbert's patronage of Mont-aux-Malades was overseen by Henry II. In the late twelfth or early thirteenth century, Alix's son, John de Préaux, reconfirmed his grandfather's grant to Mont-aux-Malades, revealing that three generations of this family supported the *leprosarium*.[88] The fact that John de Hodenc's gift consisted of land at Rouen, and favoured two of the city's monastic houses, indicates that this family had strong interests at Rouen. Another important Rouen family, the d'Esneval barons, also formed a connection to the leper house in this period. Between 1174 and 1200, Ralph and William d'Esneval pledged to deliver an annual rent of 20 *sous* to Mont-aux-Malades on the anniversary of their mother's death. Two more brothers, Renaud de Pavilly and Walter, witnessed the charter.[89] The d'Esneval were a leading family in the *bailliage* of Rouen, enjoying the title of *vidames* of Normandy and sitting at the Norman Exchequer.[90] William's contribution of 10 *sous* was to be drawn from his English revenues, testifying to the family's cross-Channel possessions and conferrring an English financial interest on Mont-aux-Malades.[91] Although members of the family were buried at the abbey of La Trinité-du-Mont, Rouen, according to Langlois it was customary for Mont-aux-Malades to host the funeral procession for one night.[92]

Rouen's archbishops and secular clergy formed an integral part of the city's aristocratic elite and, as one would expect, they also supported the leper house.[93] The act of Roscelin, son of Clarembaud, establishing a parish church at Mont-aux-Malades was confirmed by Hugh of Amiens, archbishop of Rouen, who also ratified the grant of an area of land known as Le Mont-Robert, immediately east of the leper house, by William Baril between 1130 and 1164.[94] According to Langlois, a *villa* for leisure activities was built on

[86] Appendix 2, no. 44.

[87] Ibid. no. 6.

[88] Ibid. no. 50. See also Arnoux, 'Les Origines', 146.

[89] Appendix 2, no. 77; Langlois, *Histoire*, 93, 101.

[90] Farin, *Histoire*, i/2, p. 25; Langlois, *Histoire*, 101.

[91] Appendix 2, no. 77; Langlois, *Histoire*, 101.

[92] Langlois, *Histoire*, 101.

[93] On the archbishops of Rouen see Jörg Peltzer, *Canon law, careers and conquest: episcopal elections in Normandy and Greater Anjou, c. 1140–c. 1230*, Cambridge 2008, 74–5.

[94] Appendix 2, nos 95, 105; Langlois, *Histoire*, 16. On Hugh of Amiens see Thomas G. Waldman, 'Hugh "of Amiens", archbishop of Rouen (1130–64)', unpubl. D.Phil diss. Oxford 1970. Véronique Gazeau and Thomas Waldman are currently preparing an edition of the charters of Hugh of Amiens.

this land; a later charter of May 1278 indeed mentions the '*villa* of Mont-aux-Malades'.[95] In addition, Hugh of Amiens laid down rules governing the leper house's annual fair, and was among those who requested the 1154 gift by Henry de Sully, abbot of Fécamp.[96] He also confirmed the *leprosarium's* possession of three churches, at Carville, Longpaon and Beuzeville-la-Grenier, in November 1162.[97]

Archbishop Hugh's support for Mont-aux-Malades, therefore, was indirect: rather than making gifts himself, he authorised several important donations by others. Hugh's involvement with Mont-aux-Malades reflects his strong interest in the Augustinian movement: he granted charters to almost every Augustinian house in his archdiocese.[98] Nonetheless, given the wealth of the archbishops of Rouen, it is striking that neither Hugh nor his twelfth- and thirteenth-century successors made direct donations to Mont-aux-Malades.[99] In the mid-thirteenth century Archbishop Eudes Rigaud, whose visitation records evidence considerable concern for the institutional wellbeing of *leprosaria*, did not endow Mont-aux-Malades or Salle-aux-Puelles, even though he established a leper house on his archiepiscopal manor at Aliermont in 1248, and resolved a dispute between Mont-aux-Malades and the church of Bois-Guillaume in 1253.[100]

Hugh of Amiens's successor, Rotrou of Warwick (1165–84), also offered indirect support. Between 1165 and about 1174, Rotrou renewed his predecessor's rules for the annual fair at Mont-aux-Malades.[101] Between 1165 and 1184, probably in the early 1170s, he confirmed the grant of the church at Nointot; he was also the first witness of Henry II's act making this gift.[102] Between around 1174 and 1184, he ratified a donation by Andrew de Beuze-mouchel (Bernières) of an area of land at Nointot, with the nine men who depended on it.[103] Rotrou's involvement in the 1170s, like that of Henry II, could well have been motivated by the *leprosarium's* association with Thomas Becket. Rotrou led the failed negotiations of 1170 between Becket and the king, and he was involved in arranging for Henry to receive papal absolution at Avranches in May 1170.[104] He was thus a key player in the Becket dispute and its aftermath, and, like the king, he could have patronised the

---

[95] 'villam montis leprosorum': appendix 2, no. 52(a); Langlois, *Histoire*, 16.

[96] Appendix 2, nos 33, 96(a); Langlois, *Histoire*, 12–14.

[97] Appendix 2, no. 35.

[98] Arnoux, 'Les Origines', 63.

[99] On the archbishops' wealth see Peltzer, *Canon law*, 75 and n. 6.

[100] Appendix 2, nos 19(a), 19(b).

[101] Ibid. no. 96(a).

[102] Ibid. nos 30(b), 96(b).

[103] Ibid. no. 7a; Langlois, *Histoire*, 87–8.

[104] Fournée, 'Maladreries', 127, 128; Barlow, *Thomas Becket*, 260–1.

leper house as part of a process of penance. Also in the 1170s, he dedicated the altar of the *leprosarium* chapel at Cherbourg to St Thomas, suggesting that he was participating in Becket's cult (in Normandy closely connected to leper houses) at this time.[105]

Rouen's secular clergy also supported Mont-aux-Malades. Between 1154 and 1174, probably in about 1160, Dean Geoffrey II and the chapter of Rouen confirmed the leper house's purchase of a mill at Maromme, a village immediately west of Mont-aux-Malades.[106] This was an important acquisition in the local area, consisting of both a piece of property and a resource that would enable the community to mill flour (or possibly cloth). In October 1237 Mont-aux-Malades acknowledged another gift from the dean and chapter, the right to take two loaves every day from communion at the cathedral. Presumably, this consecrated bread was distributed during mass at the *leprosarium*, and was understood to benefit the souls of those who consumed it.[107]

The early endowment of Mont-aux-Malades, promoted by the Anglo-Norman royal family, led to its establishment as a major, enduring institution. From at least the late fourteenth century, the leper house also had a special relationship with twenty-one Rouen parishes. This link was long-lasting: in February 1524 three Rouen city councillors visited the 'mallades du droit', the sick from the parishes which held rights with respect to the *leprosarium*. Two sick men from the parish of Saint-Lô and a sick woman from Notre-Dame-de-la-Ronde parish were residing at the leper house.[108] At the end of the seventeenth century, a dispute arose between the priory of Mont-aux-Malades, which by this time no longer catered for lepers, and twenty-one Rouen parishes. On 11 January 1697 these parishes claimed that, in the light of royal edicts published in December 1672 requiring *leprosaria* and hospitals no longer offering hospitality to surrender their property, Mont-aux-Malades' possessions should be used for the assistance of the poor and sick of Rouen. To legitimise their claim, the parishes argued that they had collectively founded and endowed Mont-aux-Malades in about 1131.[109] Unsurprisingly, the late seventeenth-century canons of Mont-aux-Malades did not wish to give up their property. They asserted that their institution had originated as an Augustinian priory which had initially had no hospital

---

[105] Fournée, 'Maladreries', 126–9.

[106] Appendix 2, no. 24; Langlois, *Histoire*, 16.

[107] Appendix 2, no. 11; Langlois, *Histoire*, 116.

[108] AN, Paris, S4889B, dossier 13, last document, fo. 1r. Saint-Lô and Notre-Dame-de-la Ronde were both *paroisses du Droit*: see p. 22 n. 13 above.

[109] Paris, AN, S4929–30, dossier 6: printed statement in French, 11 Jan. 1697, in which the *curés*, churchwardens and parishioners of nineteen Rouen parishes address the king and royal council regarding these matters, fos 1r–2v.

function; 'the hospitality which was subsequently extended towards lepers was only an ancillary activity'.[110] These differing perspectives underline the fact that, as is the case for many medieval *leprosaria*, the precise origins of Mont-aux-Malades are not fully understood.

---

[110] 'l'hospitalité qui s'y est depuis exercée envers les Lepreux n'y estoit qu'accessoire': ADSM, 25HP41(1): undated (late 1690s) printed paper statement, in French, issued on behalf of the prior and chapter of Mont-aux-Malades against the *curés*, churchwardens and parishioners of twenty-one Rouen parishes, 1 (fo. 1r).

2

Charity and Community
at Mont-aux-Malades

In the thirteenth century the fashion in Western Europe for Christian charity reached a peak, with the foundation and support of numerous hospitals, *leprosaria*, houses for poor women and other types of institution for the needy. Although Rouen underwent major changes in this century, following the annexation of Normandy to the French crown in 1204, Mont-aux-Malades remained a focus for high-status patronage, now receiving the support of the French royal family and household and, above all, that of Rouen's burgess elite. Initially, the involvement of members of the Anglo-Norman aristocracy also persisted. This chapter is built upon the rich documentary record for the leper house in this century, presenting a sample of material from the charters that record donations and other property transactions.[1] Mont-aux-Malades evidently became a major property holder in Rouen at this time, by virtue of which the leper community was connected to mainstream society. The charter evidence and other sources, particularly the *Register* of Eudes Rigaud, also make it possible to reconstruct the community at Mont-aux-Malades, in the thirteenth century and beyond.

Aristocratic patronage for Mont-aux-Malades in the thirteenth century

In 1204 Philip Augustus annexed Normandy to the French royal domain, and English ties with Normandy were severed.[2] Although continuity in ecclesiastical patronage was possible after 1204, as demonstrated by the gift by the dean and chapter of Rouen recorded in 1237, the close links of Mont-aux-Malades to the Anglo-Norman royal family and nobility were lost.[3] Nonetheless, some nobles continued to support the leper house after 1204, evidencing the endurance of this group's links with Rouen in spite of the new political situation. Although in theory the Anglo-Norman barons were required to choose between their Norman and English lands in 1204, many endeavoured to retain their cross-channel estates. William I Marshal

---

[1] For a more comprehensive list of the contents of charters see appendix 2 at pp. 142–81.

[2] John W. Baldwin, *The government of Philip Augustus: foundations of French royal power in the Middle Ages*, Berkeley 1986, 193–4.

[3] Appendix 2, no. 11.

(1146–1219), for example, swiftly did homage to Philip Augustus for his wife Isabelle de Clare's lordship of Longueville in the Pays de Caux. These ties continued until the 1220s when, with obstacles such as port closures and the need to obtain travel permits between England and Normandy, the remaining cross-channel aristocratic interests declined.[4]

William I Marshal's second son, Richard Marshal, later earl of Pembroke (1231–4), appears as a patron of Mont-aux-Malades in the early 1220s.[5] Following the death of his father in 1219 and that of his mother in 1220, Richard did homage for the family's Norman lands of Longueville and Orbec at the French court. From 1220 until 1231, when his brother, William II, died and Richard inherited his English lands, Richard was mainly resident in Normandy. He attained particularly high status through his marriage, by May 1223, to Gervaise, daughter of Alan de Dinan, a leading Breton baron. Richard apparently became marshal of the French royal army, indicating that the French king could even deploy members of the Anglo-Norman nobility in military service.[6]

In a charter issued at Rouen in May 1223, Richard Marshal granted the sale of a house in front of Rouen cathedral which his man Robert Lavenier had concluded with Mont-aux-Malades.[7] For the sake of his ancestors' souls, Richard gave to the prior and community a pair of fur gloves which he enjoyed as rent from the house, in return for which he expected a pair of 'single gloves' worth 3 *deniers* (current money) to be delivered annually to himself and his heirs.[8] Given Richard's assistance to Norman merchants in obtaining passage in England, and the licensing of merchants described as Richard's 'men' by Henry II (1216–72) in 1230, it is likely that Robert Lavenier was a Rouen merchant.[9] Indeed, in Robert Lavenier's own charter granting the house to Mont-aux-Malades (March 1223), he describes himself as 'citizen of Rouen', revealing that he was a member of the communal government.[10] Here there is clear evidence that the longstanding aristocracy and the emergent burgess elite intersected and were bound to each other by social ties. Richard Marshal's confirmation of his man's transaction, and his wish to conserve an aspect of his lordly privilege regarding the property, indicate that some Anglo-Norman nobles still participated actively in property transactions in post-1204 Rouen.

---

[4] Kathleen Thompson, 'L'Aristocratie anglo-normande et 1204', in Pierre Bouet and Véronique Gazeau (eds), La Normandie et l'Angleterre au moyen âge, Caen 2003, 183, 186.

[5] Appendix 2, no. 85; Daniel Power, 'The French interests of the Marshal earls of Striguil and Pembroke, 1189–1234', ANS xxv (2002), 213 n. 75.

[6] Power, 'French interests', 200, 210, 211, 213–14.

[7] Appendix 2, nos 85, 89.

[8] 'cyrothecarum singularum': ibid. no. 85.

[9] Power, 'French interests', 218, 220–1.

[10] 'Civis Rothomagi': appendix 2, no. 89.

Another, more local aristocratic family patronised Mont-aux-Malades in the 1220s. On 1 March 1220 Robert Poulain, archbishop of Rouen (1208–21), gave notice that Roger, son of Ansger de Castenay, had bequeathed half his house in the parish of Saint-Vincent, Rouen, to Mont-aux-Malades and La Madeleine hospital on the occasion of his departure for Boulogne. If Roger died there or did not return, the two religious houses were to possess this property in perpetual alms; if he came back, however, he would retain possession of it.[11] Roger may have been preparing to join a military campaign, perhaps in support of Philip Augustus in the strategically important channel county of Boulogne. French relations with Boulogne had been increasingly tense since the late twelfth century as a result of the disloyal actions of Renaud de Dammartin, count of Boulogne (1190–1227), who concluded alliances with Richard I and John of England and with the count of Flanders, and led a revolt in 1211.[12] Two witnesses of a charter of Ralph, son of Stephen for Mont-aux-Malades (February 1161) were Everard de Castenay and his grandson William, indicating that the de Castenay were a longstanding, local aristocratic family.[13] The manner in which Roger's grant favoured more than one religious house simultaneously echoes the multiple gifts made by other nobles, such as that of John de Hodenc and Alix de Préaux in the late twelfth century.[14] This suggests that Roger de Castenay was adhering to traditional patterns of aristocratic patronage, in which benefactors distributed their largesse widely, in order to accumulate the maximum number of prayers for their future salvation.[15]

Rouen's burgesses and the property interests of Mont-aux-Malades in the city

In the thirteenth century, as the involvement of the Anglo-Norman nobility with Rouen waned, the civic government (commune) established during the reign of Henry II became increasingly powerful. The municipal government was dominated by the merchant elite, and members of this elite are recognisable in charters by their qualification as 'citizen of Rouen' or 'mayor of Rouen'. Already by the last decades of the twelfth century, individuals who

---

[11] 'si predictus Rogerus apud Boloniam obierit uel de partibus illis non redierit predicte due domus medietatem predicti masagii in puram et perpetuam elemosinam possidebunt ... Si autem predictus Rogerus redierit predicta medietas eidem libere remanebit': appendix 2, no. 94.

[12] Baldwin, *Government of Philip Augustus*, 200–2, 266; Power, *The Norman frontier*, 403, 456–7.

[13] Appendix 2, no. 80.

[14] Ibid. nos 6, 44. The patronage of John de Hodenc and his wife Alix de Préaux is discussed at pp. 33–4 above.

[15] Cf. Arnoux, 'Les Origines', 146.

had accumulated wealth as traders or craftsman had joined the nobility in holding positions of the highest influence at Rouen. While some individual men stand out, such as Bernard Comin and Bartholomew Fergant, others were members of families, such as the Du Châtel, Val-Richer and Pigache lineages, that dominated the burgess elite throughout much of the thirteenth century. Religious patronage served to consolidate and further the social status of this elite, which focused particularly on supporting newer religious houses that followed the Augustinian, Grandmontine and Cistercian rules.[16] Mont-aux-Malades was a key focus for such support, and received numerous houses and rents within the city from the merchants in the thirteenth century. These donations enabled the *leprosarium* to develop valuable property interests in different areas of Rouen. By virtue of these possessions, the prior and canons themselves engaged in property transactions, buying and selling interests within the city. Although the leprous residents of Mont-aux-Malades were far from being involved in this process, the leper house's status as a player in the property market of Rouen no doubt enhanced people's awareness of the leper community. Mont-aux-Malades' property interests thus promoted the continuing connection of the lepers to mainstream society. Furthermore, the community formed relationships with specific leading citizens and families, reflecting the manner in which the transactions within charters established links, mutual interests and goodwill between parties.[17]

Many of Mont-aux-Malades' possessions were situated around Rouen's main market square, the *Vieux Marché*. The market was a very large area, at least twice the size of that occupied by the cathedral, reflecting Rouen's importance as a centre of trade. It was bordered by four parish churches (Saint-Sauveur, Saint-Michel, Saint-Georges and Saint-Éloi), while the churches of Saint-Pierre-le-Portier, Saint-Jean-sur-Renelle, Saint-André-aux-Fèvres and Saint-Vincent were also nearby. The market area was thus heavily populated, both by wealthy burgesses and by lower status merchants. It is likely that well-built stone and wooden houses stood alongside much humbler dwellings (*masures*), forming one of the focal points of commercial, social and religious life in the city. The rue Brasière ran immediately south of the western edge of the market, and the rue Cauchoise immediately north-west of its northern edge.[18]

The leper house's earliest acquisitions in the market were donated by Roscelin, son of Clarembaud, Henry II's chamberlain, as part of his endowment of the parish church of Saint-Gilles at Mont-aux-Malades (between 1154 and 1165). Roscelin granted his house and garden close to the church of Saint-Sauveur, and rent from another house that he owned in the market,

---

[16] On Rouen's burgesses see Six, 'The burgesses of Rouen', 247–78, and Sadourny, 'Les Grandes Familles', 267–78.

[17] Cf. Barbara H. Rosenwein, *To be the neighbor of Saint Peter: the social meaning of Cluny's property, 909–1049*, Ithaca, NY 1989, 4–8.

[18] Cf. Periaux, *Dictionnaire*, 102–4, 238, 507.

at that time leased to a certain Everard. The total value of Roscelin's gifts, which also included rent due from a house near *Le Donjon*, the ducal tower in the south-west corner of Rouen, constituted an sizeable annual revenue of 7 *livres*.[19]

Later, in the late twelfth or early thirteenth century, Mont-aux-Malades acquired property in the rue Brasière near the market, as an entrance gift from John Pigache, a member of the Pigache family of leading burgesses. John granted a tenement and houses in the rues Burnenc and Brasière, situated between the house of Ralph Borse and the land of Matthew Le Gros, mayor of Rouen in 1195 and 1198–1200.[20] By 1223 the leper house had another possession in this area: in this year Leiarda, daughter of Gondoin, acknowledged that she owed 5 *sous* of rent to Mont-aux-Malades from a tenement in the rue Brasière located next to the land of Alix de Cailli, Peter Luce and John Blondel.[21] Like the Le Gros, the de Cailli and Luce were prominent burgess families, confirming that this area was a focus for the property interests of the elite.

In 1193–4 or 1201–3, Prior Robert of Mont-aux-Malades granted the possessions which the community had received from John Pigache to Ralph de Cailli, mayor of Rouen, for an annual rent of 12 *sous* (usual money) and a lump sum of 50 *livres* of Anjou, and gave him permission 'to build on this land in wood or stone as it pleases him'.[22] Prior Robert also specified that Ralph could sell or mortgage the land to whomever he pleased, excepting other religious houses.[23] Perhaps, because the property had originally been donated in alms to Mont-aux-Malades, it would have been inappropriate for it to have fallen into the hands of another religious community. Perhaps also there was a degree of competition among Rouen's religious houses in terms of the acquisition of valuable property in the city.

In 1205 Mont-aux-Malades received another property interest near the *Vieux Marché* as an entrance gift. Nicholas de Puteo donated 10 *sous* of rent due from two houses in the parish of Saint-Pierre-le-Portier, Rouen, when his son Nicholas took the habit at Mont-aux-Malades. The houses were held from Nicholas de Puteo by Nicholas de Busco and his son-in-law Ralph, and were situated in front of Nicholas de Puteo's own house.[24] The fact that 5 *sous* was apparently due from each property is significant: this very small sum, also owed by Leiarda, daughter of Gondoin, to Mont-aux-Malades, was the

---

[19] Appendix 2, no. 95.
[20] Ibid. no. 92(c).
[21] Ibid. no. 53.
[22] 'hanc terram edificare de ligno uel de lapide ad libitum suum': ibid. no. 92(c).
[23] Ibid.
[24] Ibid. no. 63.

usual nominal rent paid by those purchasing property in the first part of the thirteenth century.[25]

Mont-aux-Malades also developed property interests in the western and north-western parts of Rouen in the late twelfth and thirteenth centuries. This area encompassed, to the west, the parishes of Saint-Vigor, Saint-Martin-sur-Renelle and Saint-Jean-sur-Renelle, and, to the north, those of Saint-Patrice, Saint-Godard and Saint-Laurent. It was the second main area of burgess settlement. The west of Rouen, immediately north of the *Vieux Marché*, was bordered by the Renelle river, a waterway which afforded access to the market and the river Seine, and the rue Cauchoise, which led up to the porte Cauchoise, the western gate which lay in the direction of the priory of Saint-Gervais and, beyond it, Mont-aux-Malades. The north-western edge of the city was newly settled in the late twelfth century.[26] After 1204 Philip Augustus constructed his castle at the far north-western corner of Rouen, making this zone a hub of courtly and political activity in the thirteenth century.[27]

The donation to Mont-aux-Malades of a tenement in Saint-Martin-sur-Renelle parish by Robert de Saint-Jacques and his wife Emma, in 1181–2, and the subsequent lease of this property to John d'Offranville (between 1191 and 1218, probably in 1210), testify to the affluence of this area.[28] Robert and Emma de Saint-Jacques granted their house, located on the banks of the Renelle river, for the salvation of themselves, their ancestors and benefactors, with the consent of their son Peter.[29] At the time that he leased the tenement, John d'Offranville already held land adjacent to it, meaning that he was able to increase the size, and thus the value, of his holdings in this area.[30] Unlike the grant by Robert and Emma de Saint-Jacques, the agreement made between John d'Offranville and the leper house was purely financial, containing no charitable provisions. This indicates that, to this burgess, Mont-aux-Malades was purely a fellow party in a property transaction. By the early thirteenth century, therefore, the leper house was already an established participant in Rouen's property market.

Later, Peter de Saint-Jacques continued his family's patronage relationship with Mont-aux-Malades. In July 1226 Peter and his wife Avicia donated 5 *sous* annual rent due from the parish of Saint-Patrice, Rouen, to Mont-aux-Malades, for the salvation of themselves, their benefactors and their

---

[25] Bernard Gauthiez, 'Les Maisons de Rouen, XIIe–XVIIIe siècles', *Archéologie médiévale* xxiii (1993), 141.

[26] Idem, 'Paris, un Rouen capétien?', 119.

[27] Sadourny, 'L'Époque communale', 76.

[28] Appendix 2, nos 48, 92(b), 93.

[29] Ibid. no. 93.

[30] Ibid. nos 48, 92(b), 93.

friends.[31] The specification of 5 *sous* suggests that this gift may have related to a purchase from the *leprosarium*; the property interest was located in the same zone of the city as the earlier gift by his parents. In April 1262 Mont-aux-Malades acquired another possession in this area. Agnes, wife of Ralph Le Comte, of the parish of Saint-Patrice, donated a house in this parish and two pieces of land in nearby Saint-Godard parish, for her salvation and that of her ancestors.[32] This was a substantial gift, indicating that Agnes and her husband, who consented to the donation, were wealthy burgesses of high social standing.[33] Like many other burgesses, Agnes evidently had multiple property interests in different Rouen parishes. Thus, within the geographical context of the city, the burgesses's patterns of property tenure were similar to the multiple rural estates of the twelfth-century Anglo-Norman aristocracy. As the thirteenth century progressed, Mont-aux-Malades added urban possessions to the rural lands which it had received from Henry II and his nobility in the twelfth century. This reflects changes in the locus of power in the city in the thirteenth century, as well as the urban development of Rouen and the increasing economic agency of the leper community.[34]

Patronage by the French royal family and household

While the support of Rouen's burgesses for Mont-aux-Malades increased after 1204, the Capetian kings of France were less forthcoming. More generally, they were much less actively involved in the affairs of Rouen and Normandy than the Anglo-Norman kings had been. While the Anglo-Normans had regularly held their court at Rouen, the French kings resided in Paris and managed Norman affairs indirectly by means of royal officials (*baillis*).[35] Until the latter part of the thirteenth century, the Capetians exhibited only a limited interest in Mont-aux-Malades; however, Philip III (1270–85) and Philip IV (1285–1314) granted generous possessions. Their support may have been encouraged by the patronage for Mont-aux-Malades of a French royal servant, Laurence Chamberlain, Louis IX's *panetier royal* (an official of the royal household in charge of bakers and bakeries) at Rouen.[36] The gifts of these thirteenth-century royal and aristocratic benefactors differed from those of Rouen's burgesses: the French kings and their officials donated lands

---

[31] Ibid. no. 70.

[32] Ibid. no. 2.

[33] Ibid.

[34] On the growth of Rouen in the thirteenth century see Gauthiez, 'Urban development', 40–50.

[35] Baldwin, *Government of Philip Augustus*, 221–2.

[36] Langlois, *Histoire*, 97.

and churches outside Rouen, rather than rents and properties within the city walls.

In November 1207, just over three years after gaining control of Normandy, Philip Augustus issued an act at Montargis taking Mont-aux-Malades into his protection, and confirming the leper house in its possession of all that it had held under Henry II and Richard I of England.[37] A similar confirmation had been granted by King John on 16 October 1200, suggesting that, after 1204, the community at Mont-aux-Malades had solicited this ratification from Normandy's new French lord.[38] In about 1210 Philip Augustus confirmed an alms grant of 8 *livres*, 2 *sous*, 8 *deniers* to the *leprosarium*. He simultaneously granted 40 *livres* to La Madeleine hospital, and 2 *sous* to the leprous women of Salle-aux-Puelles.[39] These different sums indicate that there was a hierarchy of charitable institutions in Rouen, in terms of their size, status and perceived importance. Also, in about 1210, the king confirmed that Mont-aux-Malades was due 60 *livres* from the *vicomté* of Rouen and half the profits from the fair of Saint-Gilles, as Henry II had established earlier.[40] Philip Augustus' successor, Louis VIII (1223–6), did not issue any charters for the leper house during his brief reign, while Louis IX (1226–70), a king renowned for his piety, merely granted a confirmation of Mont-aux-Malades' possessions towards the end of his long reign (March 1269).[41]

However, Louis IX's piety could have inspired his *panetier royal* at Rouen, Laurence Chamberlain, to patronise Mont-aux-Malades. In May 1278 Laurence granted to the leper house 5 *sous* of Tours, 5 capons of annual rent due from the parish of Saint-Jacques of Mont-aux-Malades, with half an acre of land 'between Le Tronquai and the villa of Mont-aux-Malades'.[42] These possessions were located close to Mont-aux-Malades itself. Laurence disposed of them as lord of Saint-Aignan, having been granted the fief of Saint-Aignan by Louis IX in June 1259, for an annual rent of 23 *livres* of Tours.[43] His status in the area is confirmed in a charter of July 1265, when a dispute was resolved between 'Laurence Chamberlain, lord of Saint-Aignan' and a certain Robert Carbonarium, regarding a revenue which Robert claimed from the fief.[44] In August 1289, with the consent of his wife Matilda, Laurence exchanged this fief with Mont-aux-Malades for 10 *livres* of Tours

---

[37] Appendix 2, no. 73(a); Langlois, *Histoire*, 90 (misdating Philip Augustus's act to 7 Nov. 1200).

[38] Appendix 2, no. 42; Langlois, *Histoire*, 89–90.

[39] Appendix 2, no. 73(b); *Cartulaire normand*, 33 (no. 210).

[40] Ibid. (no. 211).

[41] Appendix 2, no. 54; Langlois, *Histoire*, 95.

[42] 'Inter letronquier et villam montis leprosorum': appendix 2, no. 52(a); Langlois, *Histoire*, 97.

[43] ADSM, 25HP11/(1)(iii) (?seventeenth-century copy); Langlois, *Histoire*, 97.

[44] 'Laurentium Cambarium dominum de sancto Aniano': ADSM, 25HP11/(1)(i) (?seventeenth-century copy).

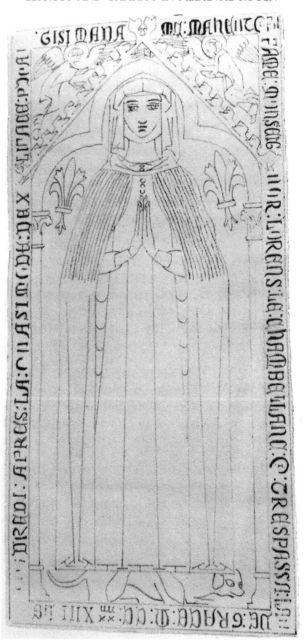

Figure 2. Tombstone of Matilda, wife of Laurence Chamberlain, now located on the left wall inside the church of Saint-Thomas at Mont-aux-Malades. Lithograph by A. Péron in Pierre Langlois, *Histoire du prieuré du Mont-aux-Malades-lès-Rouen, et correspondance du prieur de ce monastère avec Saint Thomas de Cantorbéry, 1120–1820*, Rouen 1851, facing p. 356.

annual rent and the leper house's inheritance at Sotteville (near Pont de l'Arche), Les Authieux and Pîtres.[45]

Laurence and Matilda apparently already had interests in the area of Le Pont de l'Arche: according to Pierre Langlois, they established a hospice and a night shelter for the poor at Gouy, north of Les Authieux.[46] Such philanthropic acts would suggest that the couple had charitable intentions in transacting with Mont-aux-Malades. Their close patronage relationship with the leper house is indicated by the fact that they chose to be buried there (see Figure 2).[47]

Philip III and Philip IV also supported Mont-aux-Malades in the later thirteenth century. In 1278 Philip III granted Mont-aux-Malades extensive estates at Fréville, in the Pays de Caux, for an annual rent of 180 *livres*.[48] In August 1281 the king also donated the church of Saint-Martin at Fréville, for the salvation of himself, his wife Isabelle and his father. Two priests from the leper house were to be installed in the church, one to serve as the parish priest and the other to celebrate mass there daily for the king.[49] These arrangements exemplify the manner in which some thirteenth-century benefactors arranged for their future salvation through masses and commemoration.

Philip III's grants to Mont-aux-Malades at Fréville are reminiscent of Henry II's gifts of land and church patronage at Nointot, indicating that the French kings were now taking a firmer interest in Rouen's leper house. His successor, Philip IV, made substantial grants much closer to Mont-aux-Malades, at Saint-Aignan. In September 1290, he granted the farm of Saint-Victor at Saint-Aignan, for an annual rent of 4 *livres*, 8 *sous* of Tours.[50] In December 1296 he donated the church of Saint-Aignan, for the salvation of himself and Queen Jeanne.[51] According to François Farin, the two fiefs made over to Mont-aux-Malades at Saint-Aignan, by Laurence Chamberlain and Philip IV, together constituted the entire parish.[52] As a local royal officer, Laurence Chamberlain could have encouraged the French kings to take an interest in Mont-aux-Malades. However, since Laurence held his fief at Saint-Aignan from the French king, it is equally possible that Philip IV himself had instructed Laurence's grant, as part of a wider policy to confer

---

[45] Appendix 2, no. 52(b); Langlois, *Histoire*, 97; Farin, *Histoire*, ii/6, p. 26. According to Farin, these were the lands granted to Mont-aux-Malades by the *paroisses du Droit* in 1131: see p. 22 above.

[46] Langlois, *Histoire*, 97.

[47] Ibid. 97, 356–7, 358; Deschamps, 'L'Abbé Cochet', i. 31.

[48] Appendix 2, no. 74(a); Langlois, *Histoire*, 95–6.

[49] Appendix 2, no. 74(b); Langlois, *Histoire*, 96–7.

[50] Appendix 2, no. 75(a).

[51] Ibid. no. 75(b); Langlois, *Histoire*, 98.

[52] Farin, *Histoire*, ii/6, p. 29.

royal possessions in this area on Mont-aux-Malades.[53] The estates at Saint-Aignan gave Mont-aux-Malades control of the immediate surrounding area, while the possessions at Fréville established a base approximately halfway between Rouen and its possessions at Nointot. Furthermore, both grants entitled the leper house to levy lucrative rents and feudal dues.[54] The patronage of the French crown for Mont-aux-Malades in the last quarter of the thirteenth century, therefore, resulted in the last major additions to the *leprosarium*'s patrimony.

The community at Mont-aux-Malades

The thirteenth century also marks the period from which information survives concerning the organisation of the community at Mont-aux-Malades. The *Register* of Eudes Rigaud, recording an inspection of the leper house on 29 January 1254/5, states that 'There are four communities there: one of canons, another of healthy brothers, a third of male lepers, and a fourth of female lepers.'[55] Ten years later, on 1 April 1264/5, the *Register* describes five separate groups, of canons, lay brothers, lay sisters, male lepers and female lepers.[56] Like most medieval leper houses and hospitals, therefore, Mont-aux-Malades was a mixed community, sheltering lepers and lay persons of both sexes, although there were no canonesses. Rouen's other major leper house, Salle-aux-Puelles, was very unusual in catering specifically for leprous women.

The *Register*'s word 'community' (*conventus*), also used in Mont-aux-Malades' charters to signify the whole population of the *leprosarium*, implies that the different groups were clearly distinguished from one another. Indeed, in hospitals and leper houses, men and women, and the sick and the healthy, were firmly segregated, living in separate accommodation and often following separate daily routines.[57] This resulted from the concern one would expect about chastity within a religious community, and a particular preoccupation with ensuring that religious women remained chaste. It also reflects the broader influence of concepts of enclosure and confinement upon medieval religious life.[58]

At Mont-aux-Malades, such segregation was explicitly enforced earlier in the thirteenth century by Peter de Collemezzo, archbishop of Rouen (1236–

---

[53] Langlois, *Histoire*, 98–9.

[54] Ibid. 95–6, 97; appendix 2, nos 74(a), 75(a).

[55] 'Ibi sunt quatuor conventus; unus est canonicorum, alius fratrum sanorum, tercius leprosorum, quartus leprosarum': *Regestrum*, 203; *Register*, 221–2.

[56] *Regestrum*, 513; *Register*, 585.

[57] See Hicks, *Religious life*, 101–6.

[58] See Megan Cassidy-Welch, *Imprisonment in the medieval religious imagination, c. 1150–1400*, Basingstoke 2011; Hicks, *Religious life*, ch. iii.

44). His ordinance for Mont-aux-Malades, issued in May 1237, states that '[it is] not proper or respectable that the brothers should mix with the sisters, especially the healthy with the leprous ... the prior should provide for the brothers to be separated from the sisters, and the healthy brothers and sisters from the leprous, in another cloister'.[59] The document continues: 'we wish for the two doors to the cloister of the sisters to be closed, and for the guard to be entrusted to two sisters ... one healthy and one leprous'.[60] Statutes for the mixed leper house at Sherburn, county Durham, confirmed in the early fourteenth century by Bishop Richard Kellawe (1311–16), reveal very similar arrangements. The leprous brothers and sisters occupied separate accommodation, and attended separate daily masses. They united for a shared mass on Sundays and feast days, but the statutes underline that, following this celebration, the sisters were to go back to their own accommodation, where the door would be closed.[61] Although we do not know whether Peter de Collemezzo's ordinance for Mont-aux-Malades was enacted in practice, it could describe the subsequent physical organisation of the *leprosarium* into separate male and female cloisters, subdivided into areas for the leprous and the non-leprous.

The notion that Mont-aux-Malades was divided into four distinct communities persisted: in a charter of 15 February 1330, King Philip VI of France (1328–50) referred to the four communities of Mont-aux-Malades, both healthy and leprous.[62] Another Norman *leprosarium*, the Augustinian community at Bolbec, was similarly divided into four groups, the first being priests, clerks and lay brothers, the second male lepers, the third female lepers, and the fourth healthy women and other servants.[63] Eudes Rigaud's *Register* also supplies information about the size of the community at Mont-aux-Malades.[64] On 29 January 1254/5 there were ten canons, seventeen male lepers, fifteen female lepers, and an unspecified number of lay personnel resident at Mont-aux-Malades.[65] On 8 December 1258 the community consisted of the prior, ten canons, nineteen male lepers, fifteen female lepers and sixteen healthy sisters.[66] By 1 April 1264/5 there were ten canons, five lay

---

[59] 'quia non decens audimus non honestum quod fratres cum sororibus misceantur sani maxime cum leprosis precipimus ut prior provideat quod fratres a sororibus et tam fratres quam sorores sani a leprosis que clausuram aliquam separantur': AN, Paris, S4889B, dossier 13, doc. (xxi), fo. 2r.

[60] 'Item, ad duo ostia claustri sororum clauda fieri volumus quod duabus sororibus non supportis, quarum una sana sit et alia leprosa eorum custodia commitatur': ibid.

[61] Richards, *Medieval leper*, 125.

[62] Appendix 2, no. 76(a).

[63] Hicks, *Religious life*, 99, 205.

[64] For a discussion of these figures in the *Register* see Tabuteau, 'Combien de lépreux', 19–21.

[65] *Regestrum*, 203–4; *Register*, 221–2.

[66] *Regestrum*, 325; *Register*, 371.

brothers, sixteen lay sisters, twelve male lepers and seventeen female lepers.[67] As at Sherburn, the statutes for which describe a community of sixty-five individuals, this was a relatively large community, of around sixty to seventy persons.[68] Other leper communities could be much smaller: at Bellencombre on 3 December 1255, there were four canons, five male lepers, one leprous woman, two lay sisters and four lay brothers, as well as the prior.[69] The polyptych (census) of the parish churches of the Rouen diocese drawn up in about 1240 under Peter de Collemezzo states that there were seventy parishioners at Mont-aux-Malades at this time, although it is unclear whether this refers to the leper house community, the population served by the parish church of Saint-Jacques, or indeed both.[70]

The priors and canons of Mont-aux-Malades

Other information sheds light on the respective roles of these groups and the structure of the community between the twelfth and fifteenth centuries. The priors of Mont-aux-Malades were clearly men of high status, befitting the *leprosarium's* royal connections. The first prior, Nicholas, was a friend of Thomas Becket, probably meeting him when the latter lay ill at the church of Saint-Gervais, not far from Mont-aux-Malades, in the summer of 1161.[71] Nicholas corresponded with his friend several time during his exile from England (1164–70).[72] The prior's letter of Christmas 1164, recounting his audiences with the Empress Matilda and expressing his opinions regarding the state of the English Church, identifies him as a well-informed member of the Anglo-Norman clerical elite.[73]

Much less is known about Mont-aux-Malades' subsequent priors, who may not have had such lofty connections. Nicholas's successor Herbert (*c.* 1173–90) probably served as a canon under Nicholas, and was a member of his immediate entourage.[74] He may have been Nicholas's deputy: in August

---

[67] *Regestrum*, 513; *Register*, 585.

[68] Richards, *Medieval leper*, 126.

[69] *Regestrum*, 230; *Register*, 253.

[70] 'Polyptychum Rotomagensis diœcesis', in *Recueil des historiens*, xxiii. 228, 231; *Pouillés de la province de Rouen*, ed. Auguste Longnon, Paris 1903, i–ii.

[71] Langlois, *Histoire*, 20; Barlow, *Thomas Becket*, 62; Chibnall, *Empress Matilda*, 169.

[72] Nicholas to Becket, Christmas season, 1164; before 6 July 1166; before 18 Nov. 1166; and Aug. 1167, *CTB* i. 158–69 (no. 41), 382–9 (no. 94), 548–53 (no. 113), 622–3 (no. 132). See also Becket to Nicholas, after 12 June 1166, *CTB*, i. 342–7 (no. 83), although the author of this letter was probably John of Salisbury: *The letters of John of Salisbury*, II: *The later letters (1163–1180)*, ed. and trans. W. J. Millor and C. N. L. Brooke, Oxford 1979, 64–7 (no. 157); Barlow, *Thomas Becket*, 129–30.

[73] *CTB* i. 162–9 (no. 41) at pp. 158–69; Chibnall, *Empress Matilda*, 169–71.

[74] Langlois, *Histoire*, 369.

1167 Nicholas wrote to Becket that 'if the time and opportunity should offer themselves, one of us, either myself or Master Herbert, will come to your presence as quickly as possible'.[75] In his charter granting the church of Vange, Essex, to Mont-aux-Malades, Gilbert Foliot, bishop of London, appointed 'our venerable brother Herbert, prior of the church of Saint-Jacques' to Vange.[76] This confirms that Herbert had succeeded Nicholas by the early 1170s, before the leper house's rededication to St Thomas Becket. Herbert was succeeded by Prior Robert (1191–1218), who issued at least three charters on Mont-aux-Malades' behalf.[77] John de Beuzevillette (prior 1252–88) was another long-serving prior in the thirteenth century.[78]

The prior headed a community of Augustinian canons, about which little information survives. The data supplied by the *Register* of Eudes Rigaud suggests that there was a quota of ten canons (excluding the prior) in the 1250s and 1260s, most of whom were priests.[79] When John Pigache and Nicholas de Puteo took the habit at Mont-aux-Malades around the turn of the thirteenth century, they may have joined the community as canons, although their acceptance of the habit could also mark their entry as lepers.[80] At much the same time, William, son of Bartholomew de Grand-Pont also took the habit at Mont-aux-Malades. The charter marking his entrance gift was witnessed by leading burgesses, suggesting that he was a member of this elite.[81] These men, all of high status, could have chosen to pursue a religious career at Mont-aux-Malades, perhaps being unmarried younger sons.

The laity at Mont-aux-Malades

The lay brethren formed a sizeable part of the community at Mont-aux-Malades, and played an important role in the care of the sick. The leper house was evidently a popular destination for individuals who chose to enter a religious house to fulfil pious works towards their future salvation. Membership of such a community provided them with accommodation and sustenance, and they could ultimately receive care there themselves in old age. At the ecclesiastical councils of Paris (1212) and Rouen (1214), formal legislation was laid down concerning the status of lay personnel at leper

---

[75] 'si se locus et oportunitas optulerit, quam citius fieri poterit, alter nostrum, uel ego uel magister Herebertus, uestram presentiam adibit': Nicholas to Beckett, Aug. 1167, *CTB*, i. 622–3 (no. 132).

[76] 'uenerabilem fratrem nostrum Herbertum ipsius ecclesie sancti Iacobi priorem': *The letters and charters of Gilbert Foliot*, 472 (no. 436).

[77] Appendix 2, nos 92(a), 92(b), 92(c); Langlois, *Histoire*, 369.

[78] See appendix 2, nos 41(a), 41(b).

[79] *Regestrum*, 203, 325, 513; *Register*, 221–2, 371, 585.

[80] Appendix 2, nos 63, 92(c). On John Pigache and Nicholas de Puteo see pp. 42–3 above.

[81] Appendix 2, no. 107.

houses and hospitals.[82] Lay brothers and sisters were to live according to the monastic rules of poverty, chastity and obedience, and to wear a religious habit.[83] The number of healthy lay residents in hospitals was not to exceed that of the sick and pilgrims, 'since it is more effective to have a few healthy individuals serving a large number of the sick', and since the goods donated to these institutions were intended for the use of the sick, not the healthy.[84] Married couples who joined such communities were criticised for continuing to engage in carnal activities.[85]

According to the statistics in Eudes Rigaud's *Register*, at Mont-aux-Malades in the mid-thirteenth century there was, roughly speaking, one lay individual for every two lepers (in December 1258, thirty-four lepers and sixteen lay sisters; in April 1264, twenty-nine lepers, five lay brothers and sixteen lay sisters).[86] Thus, it appears that the prescription that there should be many fewer lay brothers and sisters than sick individuals was not fulfilled at Mont-aux-Malades. Yet the presence of a large number of healthy lay persons made it possible to provide a high level of care, which would have been particularly necessary for advanced cases of leprosy. The high number of lay sisters in particular may suggest that they were responsible for nursing and other practical duties. The names of some of these women survive. In April 1233 Laurence Bouguenel granted in perpetuity the annual rent of 9 *sous* which his mother, Laurentia Bouguenel, had donated when she entered the leper house.[87] The confirmation of this grant by Laurentia's son could suggest that she was a widow, who sought both accommodation and the opportunity to fulfil pious works by joining the community. In 1296 Matilda Piguet, widow, of the parish of Saint-Gervais, Rouen, donated two pieces of land at Saint-Gervais, a piece of land at Saint-Aignan and 22 *sous* annual rent to Mont-aux-Malades, 'for the sake of God, in alms, in order to find her living there sufficiently for as long as she should live'.[88] Matilda already resided not far from Mont-aux-Malades at Saint-Gervais, and may already have been acquainted with the community.

Lay men also entered Mont-aux-Malades. By 1238 Ralph Legoix de Montigny had joined the community, donating himself and his possessions.[89] Four years previously (March 1234), Ralph and his wife Matilda had

---

[82] *Sacrorum conciliorum nova, et amplissima collectio ...*, xxii, ed. J. D. Mansi, Venice 1778, cols 835–6, 913.

[83] Ibid. col. 836.

[84] 'Cum autem pauci sani possint multis infirmis competentius ministrare': ibid.

[85] Ibid.

[86] *Regestrum*, 325, 513; *Register*, 371, 585.

[87] Appendix 2, no. 51.

[88] 'pour dieu et pour aumosne et pour trouver ly son Vivre suffisalment tant comme elle Vivra': ibid. no. 58.

[89] Ibid. no. 79; Langlois, *Histoire*, 329.

entered into a fraternity arrangement with the abbey of Saint-Georges-de-Boscherville, west of Rouen.[90] In 1238 the abbot and community of Saint-Georges gave notice that Ralph had earlier given himself and all his goods, worth 500 *livres* of Tours, to their monastery. By consequence, they required him to leave Mont-aux-Malades and return these possessions to them.[91] The very large size of this gift indicates that Ralph and Matilda were a wealthy aristocratic or burgess couple. It is possible that, between March 1234 and 1238, Matilda had died, and Ralph decided to retire to Mont-aux-Malades rather than Saint-Georges-de-Boscherville. The nature of Ralph's donation, constituting himself and all his worldly goods, distinguishes him as a *donné*, a lay person who entered into a contractual arrangement with a religious house, making over himself or herself and his or her possessions in return for the right to join the community and to make use of its resources.[92] A very similar arrangement was made at the leper house of Saint-Lazare, Paris, in June 1250, when Gila, daughter of Flora (widow of Bertaud de Termes), donated herself and her possessions to the *leprosarium*.[93] For an unknown reason, perhaps having fallen into dispute with the monks of Saint-Georges, or believing that living with lepers and supporting their care was more spiritually beneficial than joining an abbatial community, Ralph Legoix chose Mont-aux-Malades over the abbey of Saint-Georges.

The community of lepers

The population of lepers at Mont-aux-Malades was relatively stable in the mid-thirteenth century: there were thirty-two leprous residents in 1254, thirty-four in 1258 and twenty-nine in 1264.[94] Leprosy is a chronic disease, and many afflicted individuals presumably lived there for several years, if not for decades. While we only know the names of a handful of the lepers, it is clear that many were of high status, as was also the case at Saint-Lazare of Paris.[95] In his May 1237 ordinance, Archbishop Peter de Colle-

---

[90] Act of Ralph Legoix and his wife Matilda, making an alms gift to mark their acceptance into the community of Saint-Georges-de-Boscherville, Mar. 1234, BM, Rouen, MS Y52 (thirteenth-century cartulary of the abbey of Saint-Georges-de-Boscherville), fos 145r–146r, and act of the official of Rouen confirming the alms gift by Ralph and Matilda, Mar. 1234, fo. 146r–v.

[91] Appendix 2, no. 79.

[92] Charles de Miramon, *Les 'Donnés' au moyen âge: une forme de vie religieuse laïque v. 1180–v. 1500*, Paris 1999, 8.

[93] *Recueil d'actes de Saint-Lazare*, pp. xiv, 238–9 (no. 239). At Saint-Lazare, Paris, both the healthy and the leprous sometimes gave themselves and their possessions to the house: pp. xiv, 12–13 (no. 9), 24–5 (no. 19).

[94] *Regestrum*, 203–4, 325, 513; *Register*, 221–2, 371, 585.

[95] See *Recueil d'actes de Saint-Lazare*, p. xvi.

mezzo forbade the canons of Mont-aux-Malades from accepting entrance gifts on behalf of lepers.[96] This implies that, like the canons and lay brethren joining the community, prior to 1237 the lepers had to sponsor their own admission, another feature shared with Saint-Lazare of Paris.[97]

Lepers from other religious houses entered Mont-aux-Malades, revealing that high-status clerics were among the sick. Eudes Rigaud's *Register* reports that on 6 December 1258 two monks from the abbey of Saint-Wandrille, west of Rouen on the river Seine, both afflicted by leprosy, were at Mont-aux-Malades.[98] On 18 February 1297 the prior of Mont-aux-Malades, probably Prior Richard (?–1298), issued a charter outlining the provisions to be made for monks from Saint-Ouen, Rouen's largest abbey, at Mont-aux-Malades. A monk was to receive bread and wine daily from the abbey, and to have a diet of meat, eggs and herrings. He was to enjoy a pittance of food or drink whenever the canons of Mont-aux-Malades did, as if he was one of them. In addition, he had a manservant and was permitted to return to Saint-Ouen whenever he needed to.[99]

On at least one occasion, leprous brethren from Rouen's La Madeleine hospital were also accommodated at Mont-aux-Malades. In October 1261 Henry, prior of La Madeleine, issued a charter marking the entrance of two leprous members of the hospital community, Brother Roger, canon, and Sister Haisia, to Mont-aux-Malades.[100] Like the monks from Saint-Ouen, the two individuals enjoyed special treatment, having the same entitlements to food and drink as the brothers and sisters of Mont-aux-Malades.[101] Presumably, Canon Roger had the same diet as the canons, while Sister Haisia shared that of the lay sisters.

The fact that certain monastic communities elected to send their leprous members to Mont-aux-Malades distinguishes it from the other leper houses of the Rouen area, and underlines its high status. Since monasteries had their own infirmaries, and La Madeleine was a hospital for the sick, the removal of these individuals to the leper house confirms that it was considered important for lepers to enter a leper community. Nonetheless, leprous monks and nuns were accorded a higher status than the other lepers at Mont-aux-Malades, being associated more readily with the healthy members of the community than with the sick. This suggests that the social organisation of the leper house was more complex than Archbishop Rigaud's model,

---

[96]   AN, Paris, S4889B, dossier 13, doc. (xxi), fo. 1r–v; Langlois, *Histoire*, 330.

[97]   See *Recueil d'actes de Saint-Lazare*, pp. xiv–xv.

[98]   *Regestrum*, 325; *Register*, 371; Ferdinand Lot, *Études critiques sur l'abbaye de Saint-Wandrille*, Paris 1913, p. cix n. 2.

[99]   Appendix 2, no. 86; Langlois, *Histoire*, 369.

[100]   Appendix 2, no. 32; Langlois, *Histoire*, 123.

[101]   Appendix 2, no. 32.

of four or five separate groups, implies. In fact, there were many subcategories within these groups, each with their respective entitlements and duties.

Although, in 1237, Peter de Collemezzo prohibited entrance gifts, the practice was clearly revived subsequently. In 1312 Peter de Saint-Gille donated 10 *livres* of Tours and two houses in the parish of Saint-Martin-sur-Renelle, Rouen, in return for the right to be received into the community of the sick at Mont-aux-Malades for the rest of his life. Peter acted 'by the necessity of the disease with which I am taken', indicating that he was suffering, or believed to be suffering, from leprosy.[102] The nature of his donation suggests that he was very wealthy: 10 *livres* of Tours was a substantial sum, and he made over two properties in the affluent district of Saint-Martin-sur-Renelle. In 1323 John Le Vilein made a similar gift in order for his brother Laurence Le Vilein to be received as a brother at Mont-aux-Malades, and to enjoy the goods of the house 'like one of the other brothers of his condition'.[103] Another brother, Roger, now deceased, had held the status of citizen of Rouen, suggesting that this was a family of high social standing.[104] The language of both the relevant documents avoids referring explicitly to leprosy, suggesting that, for affluent families at this time, the disease was problematic and evoked stigma.

At the other end of the social spectrum, Mont-aux-Malades also catered for itinerant lepers from the late fourteenth century, if not earlier. A charter of Charles VI that refers to the leper house's link to twenty-one parishes of Rouen (18 June 1393) also states that it should receive 'all the passing sick, or those who do not have any other place [to go], wherever they come from'.[105] Since urban *leprosaria* often required entrants to be local citizens and to support their admission financially, as well as to adopt a quasi-monastic lifestyle, many more lepers lived outside institutions than within them. These wandering lepers were a recognisable social category, known in French as *lépreux forains* ('outside lepers') and in German as *Sondersiechen* ('external patients').[106] In the course of the fourteenth century, particularly following the Black Death, vagrancy became an increasingly serious problem that was associated with disorder and the transmission of disease. The presence of beggars at Rouen increased due to the upheaval of the Hundred Years' War (1337–1453): the chronicle of Pierre Cochon, for example, refers to a mad woman begging on the edge of the woods near Salle-aux-Puelles in the 1330s.[107] It is possible that Mont-aux-Malades opened its doors to passing

---

[102] 'pour la necessite de la ma[lla]die dont jestois ocupe': ibid. no. 69.

[103] 'comme un des autres freres de sa condition' : ibid. no. 46.

[104] Ibid.

[105] 'tous les malades passans ou qui nauioient autre lieu a eulx conominer de quelque partie ou pais que il soient': AN, Paris, S4889B, dossier 13, no. 14.

[106] Demaitre, *Leprosy*, 46.

[107] *Chronique normande*, 66–8.

lepers at around this time, to provide temporary shelter and, perhaps, to reduce the overall presence of wandering lepers in the roads and countryside.

By the first quarter of the sixteenth century, Mont-aux-Malades still provided for itinerant lepers. The report of an inspection of the leper house on 19 February 1524, by three city councillors of Rouen, John Le Roux, William Anbery and John du Hamel, mentions 'the hospital for the poor passing sick, which is near the church of Saint-Jacques within the enclosure'.[108] This description indicates that there was a separate building for the passing leprous close to the edge of the *leprosarium*'s grounds, in the vicinity of the former priory church of Saint-Jacques. The passing sick were thus distanced from the community proper, much as monastic prisons were often located on the edge of the precinct, but nonetheless provision was available to them. The councillors spoke to a woman, the widow of a leper, who had been in charge of this separate hospital for three or four months.[109]

The history of Mont-aux-Malades reflects the broader picture of social, religious and political change at Rouen between the central Middle Ages and the early modern period. In the thirteenth century, charity remained an important tool of the affluent, from kings to city burgesses, used to create social bonds and enhance prestige, as well as to procure the future salvation of donors and their families. Women as well as men were highly active as charitable patrons. The fact that Mont-aux-Malades catered for lepers undoubtedly made it especially attractive to benefactors. Although attitudes towards the leprous were complex, lepers were increasingly seen as a special religious group in the thirteenth century, chosen by God to suffer on earth and be saved.[110] Supporting the needs of lepers as members of a monastic community was therefore a particularly pious act.

The evidence for the internal organisation of Mont-aux-Malades confirms that this was a religious community, where non-leprous lay men and women, as well as Augustinian canons, chose to live alongside the sick. In addition, at certain points in time the lepers themselves offered entrance gifts for the privilege of joining the community. The presence of poor passing lepers, and the privileged status of leprous religious from nearby monastic houses, testify to the multiple statuses of lepers at Mont-aux-Malades, and to the many layers of community there. In the fourteenth century, at Rouen and throughout Western Europe, attitudes towards lepers became less positive, and charity for the leprous decreased. Many fewer charters for Mont-aux-Malades survive from the early 1300s onwards, but the leper house did

---

[108] 'lhospital ordonne pour les povres mallades passans Le quel est prez de lesglise de St Jacque dedens Lenclos': AN, Paris, S4889B, dossier 13, last document, fo. 1v.

[109] Ibid. fos 1v–2r.

[110] See Touati, *Maladie*, 188–200.

continue to receive gifts and to engage in property transactions with Rouen's citizens. Furthermore, despite the decline in the incidence of leprosy in the later Middle Ages, Mont-aux-Malades continued to provide for lepers in the sixteenth century.

3

Rouen's Other Leper Houses: Institutions, Gender and Status

There were several *leprosaria* around Rouen in addition to Mont-aux-Malades, as befitted a city of Rouen's size and importance. Most of these houses were small, modest foundations. Although each leper house served a distinct local community, these institutions were also interconnected, through relationships with each other and with Mont-aux-Malades. These connections suggest that provision for lepers was to some extent coordinated, not necessarily through ecclesiastical or municipal oversight, but rather through the related activities of different leper houses. The female house of Salle-aux-Puelles stands out as an institution of comparable status to Mont-aux-Malades; other *leprosaria* were considerably less wealthy and sometimes ephemeral, and have left a much fainter trace in the documentary and material record. As was the case elsewhere, in Rouen the *leprosarium* was clearly a flexible type of institution, with a variety of functions, which ranged from the facilities for diagnosis, bodily care and spiritual services at Mont-aux-Malades, to the much more basic hospitality provided by the leper houses at Darnétal, Bois-Guillaume and other villages. The diverse services offered by the *leprosaria* reflect how responses to leprosy varied and changed over time, and also highlight the multiple social statuses of sufferers.

A leper house for women[1]

The character of Salle-aux-Puelles permits an exploration of female religiosity and piety in the context of leprosy, building upon the wealth of literature on medieval religious women that has been published over the last twenty-five years.[2] Focusing on the special medical, spiritual and moral issues associated with the care of leprous women, this section describes the

---

[1] On Salle-aux-Puelles see also Elma Brenner and Bruno Tabuteau, 'La Salle-aux-Puelles, à Rouen: une léproserie de femmes', in Bruno Tabuteau (ed.), *Les Léproseries organisées au moyen âge*, *Revue de la Société Française d'Histoire des Hôpitaux* clii (2014), 44–50.

[2] See, for example, Caroline Walker Bynum, *Holy feast and holy fast: the religious significance of food to medieval women*, Berkeley 1987; Penelope D. Johnson, *Equal in monastic profession: religious women in medieval France*, Chicago 1991; Patricia Skinner, *Women in medieval Italian society, 500–1200*, Harlow 2001; Hicks, *Religious life*; and

foundation and endowment of Salle-aux-Puelles, the resident community and discipline, the physical resources and infrastructure of the *leprosarium*, and how the leprous women were cared for. It also examines the important changes that the institution underwent in the course of the fourteenth century, which place Salle-aux-Puelles in the broader context of the history of Rouen. It draws upon a much smaller body of source material than exists for Mont-aux-Malades, since only a handful of documents survive for Salle-aux-Puelles, mostly conserved in the archive of the Hôtel-Dieu (formerly La Madeleine).[3]

Like Mont-aux-Malades, Salle-aux-Puelles, at Petit-Quevilly south-west of Rouen, enjoyed royal and archiepiscopal patronage, particularly that of Henry II, who made a key donation to the community in the 1180s.[4] Also known as 'La Salle du Roi', it was another high-status institution, perhaps even more so than Mont-aux-Malades, since it apparently admitted women of aristocratic birth only, who occupied a former royal residence.[5] The language of the documents occasionally corroborates the women's distinguished status: a list of alms due from the Norman Exchequer between January 1200 and February 1205 refers to 'the leprous ladies of Quevilly', and one of the sisters, Isabel of Avènes, is referred to as a 'noble young woman' in the visitation records of Eudes Rigaud.[6] Salle-aux-Puelles was thus more exclusive than Mont-aux-Malades, particularly by the later Middle Ages when the latter was accommodating the passing sick, as well as lepers from twenty-one Rouen parishes. Salle-aux-Puelles was unique in Normandy in catering exclusively for women with leprosy. Nonetheless, there was a handful of female leper houses in England, which may have influenced the establishment of Salle-aux-Puelles, and there was another single-sex *leprosarium* in Normandy, Saint-Nicolas of Évreux, which provided specifically for leprous men.[7] Although the vast majority of *leprosaria* and hospitals in France and England accommodated both men and women, the statutes of these institutions indicate that there was, in theory at least, a strict internal segregation based on gender.[8]

There were at least four female *leprosaria* in the south of England. Henry II

Anne E. Lester, *Creating Cistercian nuns: the women's religious movement and its reform in thirteenth-century Champagne*, Ithaca, NY 2011.

[3] ADSM, H-Dépôt 1, A39, F1.

[4] Appendix 2, no. 30(i).

[5] Farin, *Histoire*, ii/5, pp. 121, 122; P. Duchemin, *Petit-Quevilly et le prieuré de Saint-Julien*, Pont-Audemer 1890, repr. Saint-Étienne-du-Rouvray 1987, 231.

[6] 'Dominabus leprosis de Chivilli': *Les Registres de Philippe Auguste, I: Texte*, ed. John W. Baldwin, Paris 1992, 183; 'domicella': *Regestrum*, 546.

[7] On Saint-Nicolas of Évreux see Tabuteau, 'Une Léproserie normande'.

[8] See, for example, 'Constitutiones Hospitalis domus leprosorum de Shirburne', trans. in Richards, *Medieval leper*, 125–8 (statutes of the *leprosarium* at Sherburn, County Durham, confirmed in the early fourteenth century), and *Statuts d'Hôtels-Dieu et de léproseries:*

was linked to two or three of these, which could suggest that he had English models in mind when he endowed Rouen's female leper house. On the outskirts of Canterbury, the *leprosarium* of St James's, Thanington, provided for twenty-five women. This house was apparently founded by a physician and member of the archiepiscopal household, Master Feramin, and soon came under the patronage of Christchurch priory.[9] At Bradley, in Wiltshire, Manasser Biset, Henry II's steward, established a house for leprous women before 1155–8 on land originally held by his wife Alice. The community was subsequently organised as an Augustinian priory dedicated to the Virgin Mary and St Matthew, and the village took on the toponym 'Maiden Bradley' in the second half of the thirteenth century, due to the presence of the leprous women. Between 1155 and 1158 Henry II confirmed the dona-tion of the churches of Kidderminster and Rockbourne by Manasser Biset to the community. Manasser had received the manor of Kidderminster from the king, and this could thus be seen as an indirect gift from the monarch.[10] There was also a community of female lepers at Woodstock, Oxfordshire, which may have been linked to Henry II. The 1181–2 pipe roll reveals that a certain Amiotus of Woodstock was paid from the revenues of the see of Lincoln for building houses for the community. Max Satchell argues that, if the building work marked the foundation of the *leprosarium*, 'Henry II could be regarded as founder as he would have authorized the payment from the vacant see.'[11]

At Westminster, outside London, a *leprosarium* dedicated to St James had been established by the reign of Henry II.[12] This institution appears to have provided specifically for leprous girls or young women (a community of either thirteen or fourteen leprous individuals).[13] Henry II issued a charter in its favour, as did King John, who confirmed the possessions of 'the leprous girls of St James outside London next to Westminster' in the fifth year of

---

recueil de textes du XIIe au XIVe siècle, ed. Léon Le Grand, Paris 1901, 224–30 (statutes of the *leprosarium* at Amiens, confirmed on 21 July 1305). See also pp. 48–9 above.

[9] Sheila Sweetinburgh, *The role of the hospital in medieval England: gift-giving and the spiritual economy*, Dublin 2004, 80; William Dugdale, *Monasticon anglicanum*, London 1817–30, vi/2, 765.

[10] Brian Kemp, 'Maiden Bradley priory, Wiltshire, and Kidderminster church, Worcestershire', in Malcolm Barber, Patricia McNulty and Peter Noble (eds), *East Anglian and other studies presented to Barbara Dodwell*, Reading Medieval Studies xi (1985), 87–9; Satchell, 'Emergence', 336. See also Sethina C. Watson, '*Fundatio, ordinatio* and *statuta*: the statutes and constitutional documents of English hospitals to 1300', unpubl. D.Phil diss. Oxford 2004, 335.

[11] Satchell, 'Emergence', 394–5.

[12] Huneycutt, *Matilda of Scotland*, 106; Marjorie B. Honeybourne, 'The leper hospitals of the London area, with an appendix on some other mediaeval hospitals of Middlesex', *Transactions of the London & Middlesex Archaeological Society* xxi (1963), 54.

[13] Kealey, *Medieval medicus*, 90; Huneycutt, *Matilda of Scotland*, 106.

his reign.[14] Henry III similarly confirmed the community's possessions, while Edward I granted it the right to hold an annual fair of four days over the feast of St James.[15] Although the exact age range signified by 'puellae' is unclear, provision for leprous girls and adolescent women would have made St James's a particularly specialised institution. There is less archaeological evidence for leprosy in children than in adults; nevertheless, young people certainly suffered from leprosy, as demonstrated by the case of King Baldwin IV of Jerusalem (1161–85), who developed leprosy as an adolescent and died at the age of twenty-three.[16] Leprous children may have been a particular focus of compassion and, given their innocence, may have challenged ideas about leprosy as a punishment for sin, immorality and promiscuity.

Although Henry II's charter for Salle-aux-Puelles refers to a community of 'women' rather than 'girls', it is still noteworthy that the house's popular name by the mid-thirteenth century was 'Aula Puellarum'.[17] Like 'maiden' in Maiden Bradley, the term *puellae* signified virginity and chastity, and this name was thus highly appropriate for a community of religious women. Yet the model of the women-only *leprosarium* also reflects anxieties about the moral and sexual conduct of leprous females. Excessive sexual activity was included among the causes of leprosy in thirteenth- and fourteenth-century medical works, and women were considered to be particularly responsible for sexual transmission.[18] It was held that leprous females infected male partners but not *vice versa*, and that a woman who had intercourse with a leprous man would transmit the disease to subsequent partners (especially her next partner) while not contracting leprosy herself. A woman's ability to pass on leprosy while remaining immune was connected to the understanding that

---

[14] For Henry II's charter see Huneycutt, *Matilda of Scotland*, 106; VCH, *A history of the county of Middlesex*, i, ed. J. S. Cockburn, H. P. F. King and K. G. T. McDonnell, London 1969, i. 206–10; VCH, *A history of the county of London*, ed. William Page, London 1909, 542–6; and 'leprosis puellis de Sancto Jacobo extra London' justa Westm': *Rotuli chartarum in turri Londinensi asservati*, I/1: (1199–1216), ed. T. Hardy, London 1837, 117. John refers to his father's charter in favour of this leper community.

[15] Dugdale, *Monasticon*, vi/2, 638.

[16] Mary E. Lewis, 'Infant and childhood leprosy: present and past', in Charlotte A. Roberts, Mary E. Lewis and Keith Manchester (eds), *The past and present of leprosy: archaeological, historical, palaeopathological and clinical approaches*, Oxford 2002, 163, 165, 166; Piers D. Mitchell, 'An evaluation of the leprosy of King Baldwin IV of Jerusalem in the context of the medieval world', in Bernard Hamilton, *The leper king and his heirs: Baldwin IV and the crusader kingdom of Jerusalem*, Cambridge 2000, 245–58.

[17] 'feminis leprosis': appendix 2, no. 30(i); *Regestrum*, 34 (visit to 'Aulam Puellarum' by Eudes Rigaud on 17 Mar. 1248/9).

[18] On women's role in transmission see, for example, the description of the infection of a bachelor of medicine by a leprous countess whom he impregnated in Bernard de Gordon's *Lilium medicinae* completed in 1305: *Practica medicinalis (Lilium medicinae)*, Wellcome Library, MS 130 (fourteenth century), fo. 18r, and *Practica seu Lilium medicinae*, Naples 1480, fos 26v–27r.

the uterus was a hard and cold organ, meaning that it retained infected semen but did not absorb it into the body.[19] These ideas credited prostitutes, who had multiple partners within a short space of time, with a key role in transmitting leprosy, thus increasing the immoral associations of women with respect to this disease.[20] While concern about the chastity of the residents of *leprosaria* related most obviously to the religious organisation of these communities, in some instances it could also have been informed by ideas about leprosy and sex. The perceived need to prevent leprous women in particular from engaging in sex may have motivated the foundation of the female *leprosaria* in England and Normandy, where they would be isolated from contact with men.

The foundation and endowment of Salle-aux-Puelles

Although it is unknown precisely when the community of leprous women at Petit-Quevilly was established, it does appear to have already been in place at the time of Henry II's gift in the 1180s.[21] Between April 1185 and January 1188, for his own salvation and that of his ancestors and his successors, the king donated an enclosure of houses at Quevilly, along with an income of 200 *livres* of Anjou per year from the *vicomté* of Rouen, 'to the leprous women of Quevilly'.[22] The money was intended to provide for the women's sustenance and clothing, until the king was able to locate another source of income. He also granted them the meadow of Quevilly, the right to put their animals to pasture in the nearby forest of Rouvray, and the right to take wood from the forest to heat and repair their houses.[23] Salle-aux-Puelles continued to receive the generous sum of 200 *livres* annually after 1204 when the obligation to pay it passed to the French kings: the sum is included in a list of alms payable from the Norman Exchequer between January 1200 and February 1205, and it is mentioned in the *Register* of Eudes Rigaud at December 1258.[24]

According to Dudo of Saint-Quentin, there had been a ducal *villa* at Quevilly, on the other side of the Seine from Rouen, since the time of

---

[19] Demaitre, *Leprosy*, 171–4; Danielle Jacquart and Claude Thomasset, *Sexuality and medicine in the Middle Ages*, trans. Matthew Adamson, Cambridge 1988, 185–90.

[20] Jacquart and Thomasset, *Sexuality and medicine*, 190.

[21] Duchemin, *Petit-Quevilly*, 226–30.

[22] 'feminis leprosis de Quevilli': appendix 2, no. 30(i), quoted here from *Recueil des actes de Henri II, roi d'Angleterre et duc de Normandie*, ed. Léopold Delisle and Élie Berger, Paris 1909–27, ii. 297 (no. 678).

[23] Appendix 2, no. 30(i).

[24] *Les Registres de Philippe Auguste*, 183; *Regestrum*, 325; *Register*, 372 (mistranslated as 'five hundred pounds annually').

William I Longsword (d. 942); this became a major royal residence under Henry I.[25] The abbey of Bec-Hellouin held the lordship of Quevilly as part of its original endowment of the 1030s.[26] In about 1161 Henry II undertook building work on the site of the ducal residence: Robert of Torigni tells us that 'he made a park and a royal residence within the palisade at Quevilly'.[27] The works took place at a time when the king was engaged in a number of construction works: Torigni states that Henry also built the *leprosarium* near Caen, improved most of his castles on the Norman frontier, and undertook building work on other castles and royal manors in Normandy and elsewhere in this year.[28] The residence at Quevilly may well have been occupied by the Empress Matilda during the last years of her life prior to her death in 1167, a period when she was closely connected with the priory of Notre-Dame-du-Pré, also on the south side of the Seine.[29] From the 1170s, however, given Henry II's increasingly long absences from Rouen, the manor may have been largely unoccupied, although the king issued two charters for Mont-aux-Malades from Quevilly during that decade.[30] This lack of use may explain the king's decision to grant the residence to the leprous women of Quevilly in the 1180s; he had already made a similar donation in the 1170s when he granted the royal manor of Sainte-Vaubourg, on the edge of the forest of Roumare, to a group of Templars.[31] The gift of a little-used royal residence may have been a useful means of fulfilling religious patronage, as well as, perhaps, saving money. Given the empress's connection with the south side of the Seine, Henry II's endowment of Salle-aux-Puelles may also have formed part of his arrangements for his mother's soul following her death, when, according to Torigni, 'her dutiful son distributed infinite treasures to churches, monasteries, lepers and other paupers for the sake of her soul'.[32] Like his patronage for Mont-aux-Malades, Henry II's donation to the leprous women could also be interpreted as part of his penance for Thomas Becket's

---

[25] Madeline, 'Rouen', 68; 'The "Draco Normannicus" of Etienne of Rouen', in *Chronicles of the reigns of Stephen, Henry II and Richard I*, ii, ed. Richard Howlett, London 1885, 713; Chibnall, *Empress Matilda*, 151.

[26] Duchemin, *Petit-Quevilly*, 8.

[27] 'parcum et mansionem regiam fecit circa fustes plantatos apud Chivilleium': *Chronique de Robert de Torigni*, i. 331. Here 'circa' is translated as 'within', as it makes sense for the royal manor to be enclosed within a palisade, particularly given the wording of Henry II's charter for the leprous women. See also Neil Stratford, 'The wall-paintings of the Petit-Quevilly', in Stratford, *Medieval art, architecture and archaeology*, 50.

[28] *Chronique de Robert de Torigni*, i. 331–2.

[29] Chibnall, *Empress Matilda*, 151; Madeline, 'Rouen', 69.

[30] Appendix 2, nos 30(d), 30(e).

[31] Madeline, 'Rouen', 69, and 'La Politique de construction des Plantagenêt et la formation d'un territoire politique (1154–1216)', unpubl. PhD diss. LAMOP/Université Paris I 2009, i. 254; Michel Miguet, *Templiers et hospitaliers en Normandie*, Paris 1995, 403.

[32] 'Thesauros infinitos pius filius distribuit ecclesiis, monasteriis, leprosis et aliis pauperibus pro anima illius': *Chronique de Robert de Torigni*, i. 367.

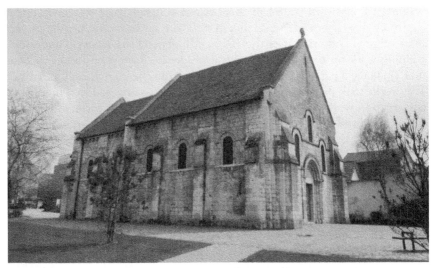

Figure 3. The chapel of Saint-Julien at Petit-Quevilly.

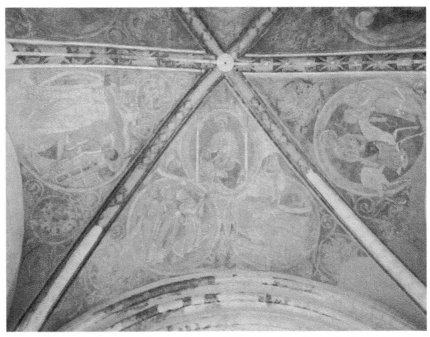

Figure 4. Wall-paintings of the infancy of Christ in the rib-vault above the choir bay, chapel of Saint-Julien at Petit-Quevilly.

murder after 1170, as well as part of his provisions for his soul at this later stage of his life.

Henry II's charter of 1185–8 states that 'I have given ... to the leprous women of Quevilly my enclosure of houses at Quevilly, where I built their residence.'[33] The 'enclosure' here is very probably synonymous with the palisade mentioned by Torigni, indicating that Henry II granted his entire manor at Quevilly to the female lepers. The reference to 'their residence' suggests that the community was already occupying the site. A chapel (see Figure 3) had been built as part of the construction works of the early 1160s, and it is still standing today, not far from the Rouen Métro stop called 'Saint-Julien'. The chapel of Saint-Julien is well-known for its twelfth-century wall-paintings, which comprise ten medallions depicting the Infancy of Christ that span the sexpartite rib-vault above the choir bay (see Figure 4).[34] The paintings were executed in the 1160s, meaning that the chapel was not decorated for the benefit of the leprous women, since the community at Quevilly was not established until two decades later.[35] Nonetheless, they may reflect a female perspective, that of the Empress Matilda.[36]

The 1180 pipe roll recording royal payments from the Norman Exchequer lists a grant worth 10 livres, consisting of one measure of wheat, four measures of wine and 1,000 herrings, 'to the chaplain of the chapel of Quevilly'.[37] The grant marks the king's endowment of religious worship in his chapel prior to its cession to the leprous women: both the wheat and the wine were to be put towards the celebration of the eucharist there.[38] In the 1180s Pope Lucius III (1181–5) issued a bull confirming the leper community's possessions and taking it under his protection, perhaps soon after the donation of Henry II. The bull implies that the community's chapel was dedicated to the Virgin Mary at this time, suggesting that the royal chapel was originally so

---

[33] 'Sciatis me dedisse ... feminis leprosis de Quevilli clausum meum domorum mearum de Quevilli, ubi mansionem suam construxi': appendix 2, no. 30(i) (quoted here from Recueil des actes de Henri II, ii. 297 [no. 678]).

[34] On the chapel of Saint-Julien see Stratford, 'Wall-paintings', and 'Le Petit-Quevilly, peintures murales de la chapelle Saint-Julien', in Congrès Archéologique de France, 161e session 2003: Rouen et Pays de Caux, Paris 2005, 133–46, and Claire Étienne-Steiner, La Chapelle Saint-Julien du Petit-Quevilly, Rouen 1991.

[35] Stratford, 'Wall-paintings', 51, 54–6.

[36] See Chibnall, Empress Matilda, 188.

[37] 'capellano capelle de Keuilleio': Pipe rolls of the Exchequer of Normandy for the reign of Henry II 1180 and 1184, ed. Vincent Moss, London 2004, 50. Duchemin states that King John donated a measure of wheat, 3 measures of wine and 1,000 herrings to the chaplain at Salle-aux-Puelles: Petit-Quevilly, 231. It has not been possible to corroborate this claim, although it is possible that John reconfirmed his father's earlier grant. I am very grateful to Paul Webster for directing me to this entry in the 1180 pipe roll.

[38] 'Pro j summa frumenti ad hostias faciendas et pro iij modiis vini ad missas cantandas': Pipe rolls, 50.

dedicated.[39] It was dedicated to St Julian, a popular patron of leper houses, by the time of the donation of Salle-aux-Puelles to Rouen's La Madeleine hospital in 1366. La Madeleine's fifteenth-century memorial book, when marking this gift, refers to 'the church of Saint-Julien of Salle-aux-Puelles, long ago called Sainte-Marie of Quevilly'.[40]

Henry II's successor Richard I (1189–99) also supported Salle-aux-Puelles. At Bec-Hellouin, on 4 April 1195, Richard donated the church of (Saint-Martin du) Grand-Couronne, a village southwest of Salle-aux-Puelles, to the leprous women, for his salvation and that of his father, ancestors and successors.[41] Given that the abbey of Bec-Hellouin held the lordship of Quevilly where Salle-aux-Puelles was situated, the location for Richard's act was no doubt significant. Although Richard apparently made no donations to Mont-aux-Malades, he was a generous benefactor to La Madeleine hospital, indicating that he did take an interest in the sick and needy of Rouen.[42] He may have associated Salle-aux-Puelles with the pious wishes of his father, who had endowed the female community in the final years of his life.

A charter of Walter of Coutances, archbishop of Rouen (1184–1207), which must have been issued in 1198–9, granted the church of Grand-Couronne to the community at the king's request. The leprous women were to come into possession of the church after the death of Robert of Saint-Nicolas, canon of Rouen cathedral, who was at that time appointed to the church. Until then, Robert of Saint-Nicolas would give a bezant of annual rent to the leprous sisters.[43] Robert was a chaplain and scribe at the cathedral in the 1190s and early 1200s, and canon from at least 1201 until at least 1214, followed by a period as chanter between 1223 and 1225.[44] He died in 1225 or later, meaning that it was a number of years before Salle-aux-Puelles took full possession of this church. François Farin cites a charter in which Roger Deshays, his wife Jeanne, his brother Stephen and his son William donated

---

[39] Farin, Histoire, ii/5, p. 122; Duchemin, Petit-Quevilly, 231.

[40] 'ecclesiam Sancti Juliani de aula puellarum quam antiquitus beate marie de Quevilly nuncupatur': BM, Rouen, MS Y42, fo. 50v.

[41] Appendix 2, no. 83.

[42] Richard's gifts to La Madeleine, which included two churches (Bénonville and Vatetot), are listed in its fifteenth-century memorial book: BM, Rouen, MS Y42, fo. 21v. See also Catherine Dubois, 'Les Rouennais face à la mort au XVe siècle, d'après l'obituaire du prieuré de la Madeleine', unpubl. MA diss. Rouen 1990, 29, 149.

[43] Farin, Histoire, ii/5 p. 122; Duchemin, Petit-Quevilly, 231. Robert of Saint-Nicolas had received life tenure of the church of Grand-Couronne from Archbishop Walter between September 1188 and July 1189: Peter A. Poggioli, 'From politician to prelate: the career of Walter of Coutances, archbishop of Rouen, 1184–1207', unpubl. PhD diss. Johns Hopkins 1984, 357.

[44] David S. Spear, The personnel of the Norman cathedrals during the ducal period, 911–1204, London 2006, 227, 229, 260; Vincent Tabbagh, Fasti ecclesiae gallicanae: répertoire prosopographique des évêques, dignitaires et chanoines de France de 1200 à 1500, II: Diocèse de Rouen, Turnhout 1998, 360; Poggioli, 'Politician to prelate', 357.

the tithes of Grand-Couronne, their part of the *pré de l'Epine* and some cultivable land in the parish.[45] As was the case with Mont-aux-Malades, the local aristocracy at Grand-Couronne may have been encouraged to support Salle-aux-Puelles by the example of the English king. Like the possessions that Mont-aux-Malades held near its parish churches at Saint-Aignan and Fréville, the accumulation of holdings at Grand-Couronne strengthened the influence that Salle-aux-Puelles could exert in this particular area.

The community at Salle-aux-Puelles was granted the right to have a priest, to administer the sacraments and celebrate mass, by Pope Lucius III in 1183, a few years after the decree of the Third Lateran Council (1179) that all leper communities should have their own priest, church and cemetery.[46] Lucius' bull also extended his protection over Salle-aux-Puelles and confirmed the community in the possessions donated by Henry II.[47] In the thirteenth century another papal bull was issued for Salle-aux-Puelles, by Honorius III (1216–27). In June 1219, in response to the petitions of the prioress and sisters of Salle-aux-Puelles, Honorius III forbade anyone from demanding tithes from them for their gardens and orchards.[48] This intervention was in line with Canon 23 of the Third Lateran Council, which stated that leper communities 'should not be compelled to pay tithes for their gardens or the pasture of animals', and confirms that Salle-aux-Puelles was considered by the Church to be a properly constituted *leprosarium*.[49] In practice, however, Salle-aux-Puelles and other leper communities could face difficulties in asserting the rights accorded to them in 1179. Here, the Salle-aux-Puelles community had needed to ask the pope to intervene to enforce its exemption from paying tithes.

While the Anglo-Norman kings and the popes supported Salle-aux-Puelles, it is less clear whether it was a focus for the charity of the kings of France after 1204 and the citizens of Rouen, the latter being the major benefactors of Mont-aux-Malades in the thirteenth century. In a general distribution of alms in about 1210 Philip Augustus (1180–1223) granted only 2 *sous* to Salle-aux-Puelles, in contrast to the much larger sums of 8 *livres*, 2 *sous*, 8 *deniers* to Mont-aux-Malades and 40 *livres* to La Madeleine.[50] Salle-aux-Puelles was much smaller than its counterparts; yet its very minor share in the royal alms is still noticeable. Of two early fourteenth-century

---

[45] Farin, *Histoire*, ii/5, p. 122; Duchemin, *Petit-Quevilly*, 231. I have not been able to locate this charter, which presumably dates from the end of the twelfth or beginning of the thirteenth century.

[46] Farin, *Histoire*, ii/5, p. 122; Duchemin, *Petit-Quevilly*, 231. I have not been able to locate this papal bull. For the 1179 decree see *Decrees of the ecumenical councils*, i. 222.

[47] Farin, *Histoire*, ii/5, p. 122; Duchemin, *Petit-Quevilly*, 231.

[48] Appendix 2, no. 34; Farin, *Histoire*, ii/5, pp. 122–3.

[49] 'de hortis et nutrimentis animalium suorum, decimas tribuere non cogantur': *Decrees of the ecumenical councils*, i. 223.

[50] Appendix 2, no. 73(b); *Cartulaire normand*, 33 (no. 210).

testaments which named many hospitals and *leprosaria* in the Rouen area as beneficiaries, only one remembered Salle-aux-Puelles. The testament of John Hardi (1304) bequeathed 10 *sous* to Salle-aux-Puelles (as opposed to 20 *sous* to Mont-aux-Malades), but that of Geoffrey Le Cras (1302) did not include Salle-aux-Puelles among its beneficiaries, while remembering Mont-aux-Malades and La Madeleine.[51]

There is evidence of very few benefactions to Salle-aux-Puelles outside the royal and ecclesiastical spheres. According to Farin, at an early date, probably in the late twelfth century, Cecily, daughter of John Fournier, gave all of her possessions to the *leprosarium* with her father's consent.[52] This may well have been an entrance gift, marking the moment that Cecily joined the community as a leprous sister or a non-leprous lay sister. In the thirteenth century there is a striking lack of evidence for gifts by Rouen's burgesses. Given the support of the burgess community for the wide spectrum of religious houses at Rouen, it is likely that a body of charters for Salle-aux-Puelles, or one or more cartularies, have been lost. Perhaps documents were discarded at the time of the leper house's unification with La Madeleine, with only certain key property deeds, such as those relating to Salle-aux-Puelles' dependent church at Moulineaux, retained. It is also possible, though perhaps unlikely, that the exclusive entrance criteria of the female leper house deterred donations.

By at least 1240 Salle-aux-Puelles had acquired the patronage of another church in the area of Grand-Couronne, namely Saint-Jacques of Moulineaux.[53] Originally a chapel, it was formally made into a parish church by Peter de Collemezzo, archbishop of Rouen, in September 1240. The aim was to provide local people in Moulineaux with a church that was accessible, since flooding meant that there were problems of access to the nearby parish churches of Sahurs and Grand-Couronne.[54] Hugh of Sahurs, already rector of the chapel at Moulineaux, was made the parish priest, at the request of the prior and community of Salle-aux-Puelles.[55] Archbishop Peter used the occasion to instruct the dean of Rouen to make an inventory of the church's books, revenues, vestments and ornaments.[56] Such possessions held by the church at Moulineaux would have been a potential source of wealth and income for Salle-aux-Puelles.

---

[51] Appendix 2, nos 26, 43.

[52] Farin, *Histoire*, ii/5, p. 122; Duchemin, *Petit-Quevilly*, 231. I have not been able to locate the charter to which Farin refers.

[53] According to Fournée, Saint-Jacques of Moulineaux was granted to Salle-aux-Puelles by Henry II: 'Les Maladreries', 106. However it has not been possible to trace any documentary evidence for this gift.

[54] Appendix 2, no. 67(b).

[55] Ibid. nos 38, 67(a).

[56] Ibid. no. 67(a).

In statutes for Salle-aux-Puelles that Eudes Rigaud drew up in August 1249, he instructed the prior to conserve fragments of food 'for poor lepers from outside'.[57] According to Eudes's *Register*, on 11 February 1265 (= 1266) the community was conserving the vestiges of its food for a female leper at Moulineaux.[58] Such an act of charity suggests that, as patron of the parish church at Moulineaux, the community at Salle-aux-Puelles took responsibility for the leprous, and perhaps other needy people, in the village. Giving away surplus food was a key marker of aristocratic status in this period, and was thus an appropriate act by the women of Salle-aux-Puelles.[59] There was apparently a small *leprosarium* at Moulineaux itself, dedicated to St Mark, where the woman may have resided.[60]

The community at Salle-aux-Puelles: piety, discipline and the care of the sick

Almost all of the available knowledge about the community and internal life of Salle-aux-Puelles is derived from a twenty-year period, 1249 to 1269, when Archbishop Eudes Rigaud periodically visited the *leprosarium*. Although it cannot be assumed that the community's organisation and circumstances were exactly the same in the decades before and after the archbishop's inspections, Eudes Rigaud's *Register* sheds much light on what life was like at Salle-aux-Puelles in the mid-thirteenth century. This was a smaller community than Mont-aux-Malades: in December 1258, there were ten leprous sisters and one 'healthy' sister, while by February 1266 there were only six leprous sisters, one of whom claimed to be healthy (perhaps, this was the same woman as in 1258).[61] Presumably, four leprous sisters had died in the intervening period, though there could have been more deaths, as well as some new arrivals. Salle-aux-Puelles was clearly organised as a priory, yet there is no explicit evidence of the rule followed by the community. Given the predominant role of the Augustinians in regulating hospitals and *leprosaria* in the twelfth and thirteenth centuries, including Mont-aux-Malades and La Madeleine at Rouen, it is possible that Salle-aux-Puelles was an Augustinian community, although Eudes Rigaud's *Register* mentions no canons or canonesses there.

According to Rigaud's statutes for Salle-aux-Puelles, promulgated in August 1249, when he had visited in April that year there had been a prior, prioress, sisters and 'other persons' at the *leprosarium*; the ordinance

---

[57] 'pauperibus leprosis extraneis': *Regestrum*, 101; *Register*, 116.

[58] *Regestrum*, 538; *Register*, 615.

[59] See Bynum, *Holy feast*, 2.

[60] Fournée, 'Les Maladreries', 106.

[61] *Regestrum*, 325, 538; *Register*, 371, 614.

prescribed that there should be a few clerics there and two or three maid-servants.[62] Thus, several non-leprous individuals played an important role in the community, and these included men. The *Register* describes the prior's role as 'the governor and administrator of all the goods of the house', indi-cating his overall authority and financial responsibility.[63] At the time of the visitations, Prior Willard was in office. He appears to have been a member of Eudes's household, occasionally undertaking inspections elsewhere on the archbishop's behalf. In September 1258 and August 1263, for example, when the archbishop was visiting various institutions at Gournay, Willard visited the local *leprosarium* of Saint-Aubin, perhaps because he was consid-ered to have special expertise regarding communities of lepers.[64] Willard's proximity to the archbishop is reminiscent of the friendship between Prior Nicholas of Mont-aux-Malades and Thomas Becket in the twelfth century, a comparison which underlines the fact that both Mont-aux-Malades and Salle-aux-Puelles were high-status institutions. In 1266 a priest, Robert, and three maidservants were at Salle-aux-Puelles.[65]

The fact that Eudes Rigaud issued statutes for Salle-aux-Puelles, 'having found the same place worthy of correction and reform, in both spiritual and temporal matters', may indicate that he was concerned about religious discipline and behaviour there.[66] A number of years later, on 11 February 1266, Eudes found strong evidence of immoral conduct: one of the sisters at Salle-aux-Puelles, Isabel of Avènes, had borne a child by Peter of Couronne, a priest.[67] The entry for 22 May 1266 reveals that Peter was the chaplain of the *leprosarium* at 'Quercu Canuta', which means that this transgres-sion involved members of two different leper communities, both of whom should have been living chastely.[68] Peter may have been a native of Grand-Couronne, where Salle-aux-Puelles held the patronage of the church. The sexual relations between Peter and Isabel indicate that the residents of Salle-aux-Puelles came into contact with people from outside the community, either within or beyond the walls. Isabel was technically counted among the leprous sisters, but 'she said that she was healthy, ... and she said that she wished to complete her time there since she was healthy, especially since, according to the tenor and custom of the law of the same place, none but

---

[62] *Regestrum*, 101, 102; *Register*, 115, 117.

[63] 'procurator et amministrator omnium bonorum dicte domus': *Regestrum*, 325.

[64] *Regestrum*, 319, 466; *Register*, 364–5, 531. On Eudes Rigaud's household see Adam J. Davis, *The holy bureaucrat: Eudes Rigaud and religious reform in thirteenth-century Normandy*, Ithaca, NY 2006, 34–7.

[65] *Regestrum*, 538; *Register*, 614–15.

[66] 'invenissemus ibidem, tam in spiritualibus quam temporalibus, correctione et reformacione digna': *Regestrum*, 101.

[67] *Regestrum*, 538; *Register*, 614.

[68] *Regestrum*, 546; *Register*, 624. In *Register* 'Quercu Canuta' is translated as 'Quesne-Canu', but it has not been possible to identify it.

leprous sisters should be in the house'.[69] The reference here to 'custom' may suggest that there was an ordinance for Salle-aux-Puelles which predated that of Eudes Rigaud and laid down its specific function as a *leprosarium* for women. Alternatively, Henry II's gift to 'the leprous women of Quevilly' itself perhaps represented this custom. The fact that Isabel had been able to bear a child strongly indicates that she was not suffering from leprosy. She could have been misdiagnosed at an earlier date, or she could previously have had the tuberculoid form of leprosy, which often recedes.[70] Indeed, Isabel could have been sent to Salle-aux-Puelles as a child. Children often exhibit tuberculoid leprosy, and she is referred to as a 'domicella', a 'noble young lady', in 1266.[71]

We gain the impression that Isabel used persuasive language to argue her case for leaving Salle-aux-Puelles, suggesting that she perceived motherhood as an opportunity to be freed from the *leprosarium*. At the same time, however, the tone of the *Register* indicates that the archbishop would in any case have required her to leave: 'we ordered her to be sent back to her father and utterly removed from there'.[72] The woman's presence set a very bad example to the other sisters. Furthermore, if the infant was still with her, it was inappropriate for an illegitimate child to be raised in a *leprosarium*. The *Register* refers to Isabel's circumstances as a 'disgrace' and a 'crime', making it clear that she had seriously transgressed, perhaps not only in terms of her religious status but also with respect to her high social status.[73] Nonetheless, it does not appear that she was excommunicated, unlike, for example, Agnes de Merla, who fled from the Cistercian nunnery of L'Abbaye Blanche in Mortain in 1232, 'abandoning her habit and returning to debauchery (*vomitus*)'.[74]

A few months later, in May 1266, Eudes Rigaud brought Peter of Couronne before him to answer for his incontinence. The *Register* states that

> He denied the scandal, but recognised its existence; and then we instructed him to make purgation on account of this with the sixth hand of priests. For making this purgation we assigned him a day in the octave of the nativity of

---

[69] 'se sanam esse dicebat, ... et dicebat se velle exigere cum esset sana, maxime cum non nisi leprose sorores iuxta tenorem privilegii cuiusdam et loco consuetudinem debeant esse in domo predicta': *Regestrum*, 538; *Register*, 614.

[70] Marcovitch, *Black's medical dictionary*, 406.

[71] Lewis, 'Infant and childhood leprosy', pp. 163–70; *Regestrum*, 546; *Register*, 624.

[72] 'eam remitti precepimus ad patrem suum et abinde penitus amoveri': *Regestrum*, 538; *Register*, 614.

[73] 'turpitudinem et scelus dicte Ysabelle': *Regestrum*, 538; *Register*, 614–15.

[74] Leonie V. Hicks, 'Exclusion as exile: spiritual punishment and physical illness in Normandy c. 1050–1300', in Laura Napran and Elisabeth van Houts (eds), *Exile in the Middle Ages: selected proceedings from the International Medieval Congress, University of Leeds, 8–11 July 2002*, Turnhout 2004, 148.

St John the Baptist, or the day after the said octave, if that is a day of rest, in the presence of us or our official of Rouen.[75]

Thus, while Isabel of Avènes left the community at Salle-aux-Puelles, Peter of Couronne underwent canonical purgation before the archbishop or his official, with six priests acting as witnesses to his good character.[76] While Isabel's crime was undeniable since she had borne a child, as a man, Peter's involvement could only be ascribed through accusation, which he denied.

As well as marking an instance of scandal and incontinence at Salle-aux-Puelles, the case of Isabel of Avènes suggests that there could be considerable solidarity, loyalty and support within a community of leprous women, since the sisters 'had concealed' the woman's crime and resultant pregnancy.[77] It is possible that Isabel's child was born and baptised at the *leprosarium*: at the nunnery of Saint-Saëns (north-east of Rouen) in 1259 the nun Nicola of Rouen gave birth inside the monastery, with two village midwives in attendance, and had her child baptised there.[78] At the time of the birth of Isabel's child, the prior of Salle-aux-Puelles was Willard. Perhaps, he had not known about this sister's pregnancy. Eudes Rigaud ordered Willard to punish the sisters and impose penance on them for their complicity, thereby underlining the fact that transgression by an individual member had broader implications for the leper community as a whole.[79]

Buildings, resources and infrastructure

Eudes Rigaud's *Register* also sheds light on the buildings at Salle-aux-Puelles and the agricultural activities of the community. The account of his visit on 17 March 1248 (= 1249) refers to the cloister, the kitchen, 'workshops', the refectory and the dormitory.[80] The record for 9 December 1258 mentions the infirmary, 'lands before the gate', a grange at Quevilly and 'meadows that suffice well for the pasture of their animals for the use of the house'.[81] The meadowland and rights of pasture in the forest of Rouvray, granted by Henry II, no doubt provided the women of Salle-aux-Puelles

---

[75] 'negavit infamiam, tamen recognovit, et tunc indiximus ei purgationem super hoc faciendam manu sexta sacerdotum; super qua facienda assignavimus ei diem in octabis nativitatis Beati Johannis Baptiste, vel in crastino dictarum octabarum, si dies ipsarum esset feriata, coram nobis vel coram officiali nostro Rothomagi': *Regestrum*, 546; *Register*, 624.

[76] On the role of the official of Rouen see Davis, *Holy bureaucrat*, 39–40.

[77] 'celaverant': *Regestrum*, 538; *Register*, 615.

[78] *Regestrum*, 337–8; *Register*, 383–4; Johnson, *Equal in monastic profession*, 123.

[79] *Regestrum*, 538; *Register*, 614–15. See Hicks, 'Exclusion as exile', 146–7.

[80] 'officinas': *Regestrum*, 34; *Register*, 38–9.

[81] 'terras ante portam; … prata que eis sufficient bene pro suis animalibus pascendum ad usum domus': *Regestrum*, 325; *Register*, 371–2.

with valuable agricultural facilities. In February 1331 (=1332), Philip VI of France responded to the complaint of the prior of Salle-aux-Puelles (now termed 'master') that John Le Veneur, master of the king's forests, had been preventing the community from enjoying its use of 'an enclosed hedged area of ditches and planted trees'.[82] The hedged area was probably an area in the forest of Rouvray where Salle-aux-Puelles had exclusive rights, although the document could also refer to the enclosed area of the original royal manor of Quevilly, as described in the twelfth century by Robert of Torigni and Henry II. The community at Salle-aux-Puelles was evidently concerned to protect its agricultural resources in the first half of the fourteenth century.

The descriptions in the *Register* suggest that Salle-aux-Puelles was organised along conventional claustral lines, with the key communal structures of the cloister, dormitory, infirmary and refectory. These buildings, none of which survives, presumably adjoined the chapel of Saint-Julien. Given the high social status of the sick residents, it is possible that the dormitory mostly accommodated staff and lay brethren, and that some or all of the leprous sisters had individual rooms. Leper houses elsewhere certainly offered private accommodation, such as that at Aumône near Pontoise in the later Middle Ages, where Jehan Duquesnoy, called 'le Bourguignon', was to be provided with his own room according to a document of May 1412 marking his entry to the house.[83] The infirmary probably catered for women in the advanced stages of leprosy, offering an intensive level of care. Many of the buildings at Salle-aux-Puelles may have originated as part of the manorial complex or 'enclosure of houses at Quevilly' donated by Henry II. The grange, for example, could well have formed part of this original enclosure. Yet it would still have been necessary to adapt and convert the original structures, particularly in order to create a cloister.

Salle-aux-Puelles had workshops, even though work is not an activity necessarily associated with a community of women who were both aristocratic and sick. Those women who were very unwell would have found it difficult to complete even simple tasks, as a result of damage to their fingers and hands, blindness and overall physical weakness. Since the leprous women were also attended by maidservants, it appears unlikely that they would have worked themselves. However, textile crafts were certainly practised by non-leprous religious women. On visiting the distinguished Benedictine abbey of Saint-Amand, Rouen, in December 1258, Eudes Rigaud prohibited the nuns from giving away 'alms-bags, frill-collars, cushions, or other such things' without the abbess's permission.[84] It is likely that the nuns of Saint-Amand, who also had maidservants, were sewing and embroidering these items, possibly in

---

[82] 'une haie close de fosses et darbres plantes': appendix 2, no. 76(b). John Le Veneur had also attacked Mont-aux-Malades's rights in the forest of Lyons: appendix 2, no. 76(a).

[83] See ch. 1 n. 17.

[84] 'elemosinarias, fresellas, vel aurarias, vel aliquid tale': *Regestrum*, 326; *Register*, 373.

their leisure time. Perhaps, at Salle-aux-Puelles, those sisters who were not too sick engaged in similar activities, producing items to be used internally by the community, donated to the poor or sold to generate income. Such activities had potential therapeutic value, giving the women an occupation and a sense of purpose.

In March 1249 Rigaud was concerned that: 'here and there, lay people enter the cloister, the kitchen and the workrooms, they go among the sisters and speak with them, without having obtained permission'.[85] He stipulated that the sisters must first obtain the permission of the prioress before speaking to lay people.[86] This detail, like the presence of workrooms, sheds light on daily life at Salle-aux-Puelles. Although in theory the community was enclosed, in practice there was contact with the world outside through the breaching of the leper house's boundary by members of the laity. Eudes Rigaud made a very similar complaint about the presence of lay people at the abbey of Saint-Ouen, Rouen, in 1258. The record of his visit to Saint-Ouen on 13 December states that 'Merchants and apothecaries often came there, and entered the cloister, bringing with them items to sell to the monks.'[87] He forbade this practice, indicating that at both Saint-Ouen and Salle-aux-Puelles the infiltration of an enclosed religious space by lay people from outside the community was perceived to be problematic.[88] At Saint-Ouen, the visitors brought trade into the cloister, an inappropriate activity for this location. Perhaps those lay people who visited Salle-aux-Puelles engaged in similar commercial activities with the sisters, although they could also have been the residents' family members and friends.

Salle-aux-Puelles in the later Middle Ages

On 31 August 1366 Salle-aux-Puelles, with all its rights and possessions, was donated to La Madeleine, Rouen's hospital for the sick poor, by Charles V of France.[89] The king made this gift at the beseeching of Thomas Le Tourneur, a royal clerk and canon of Rouen cathedral (1357–84).[90] Thomas had considerable influence in royal circles, serving as master of accounts and first secretary to Charles V, and acting as one of the king's executors on his

---

[85] 'seculares passim intrant claustrum, coquinam et officinas, inter sorores, et cum illis loquuntur, licencia non obtenta': *Regestrum*, 34; *Register*, 38.

[86] *Regestrum*, 34; *Register*, 39.

[87] 'Mercerii et apotecarii aliquotiens veniebant, et ingrediebantur claustrum, secum ibidem afferentes res quasdam monachis vendendas': *Regestrum*, 326; *Register*, 373.

[88] On monastic enclosure see Hicks, *Religious life*, ch. iii.

[89] Appendix 2, no. 13(a).

[90] BM, Rouen, MS Y42, fo. 31r.

death in 1380.[91] As a cathedral canon, Thomas's support for La Madeleine is unsurprising, since from its foundation in the eleventh century or earlier, the hospital was closely associated with Rouen cathedral. La Madeleine's memorial book, first compiled in the 1460s but apparently containing entries from an earlier book, reveals that Thomas also donated 100 *livres* to the hospital in his testament, provided the community with a book (*Catholicon*) 'and did many other good things for [the community]'.[92]

The impetus for the unification of Salle-aux-Puelles with La Madeleine hospital was the great financial need of the latter institution in the 1360s, following the Black Death and during the Hundred Years' War. In October 1359 the future Charles V, then duke of Normandy, had already responded to La Madeleine's needs. He granted the hospital exemption from paying taxes (*octrois*) in light of the diminution of its revenues as a result of the destruction and pillaging wrought by the enemy. He observed that, at the same time, increased numbers of 'the good people of the countryside' were taking refuge at the hospital, including those who were sick and women made pregnant by the enemy.[93] It was necessary to care for these women (presumably, in childbirth) and to feed their infants.[94]

Alongside the emergencies of plague and war, which affected large numbers of people in Rouen and the surrounding area, the needs of the leprous may have become less of a priority at this time. There may also have been fewer residents at Salle-aux-Puelles by 1366, due to the impact of plague and war, and perhaps also a decreased incidence of leprosy. The *leprosarium* was itself located in the vulnerable countryside affected by the war, and the chronicle of Pierre Cochon, discussing events taking place in the 1330s, describes, in passing, a deserted scene outside Salle-aux-Puelles, where the only person to be found was a mad woman begging at the edge of the woods.[95] Since the community at Salle-aux-Puelles was small even in the mid-thirteenth century, a further shrinkage in size could well have justified the diversion of its revenues to La Madeleine.

Yet the arrangements surrounding the royal donation of Salle-aux-Puelles to La Madeleine indicate that it was envisaged that the former would continue to function as a *leprosarium*, in terms of both the spiritual and the physical care of the sick. Charles V's donation, as recorded in La Madeleine's memorial book, specified that mass was to be celebrated in the church of Saint-Julien every Sunday, and on solemn days and feasts. Charles V's donation charter of November 1366 expressed the hope that the souls of 'the

---

[91] Tabbagh, *Fasti*, 378–9; Dubois, 'Les Rouennais', 47.

[92] 'et alia multa bona fecit nobis': BM, Rouen, MS Y42, fo. 31r; Dubois, 'Les Rouennais', 10–11, 47.

[93] 'des bonnes gens du pais': *Documents concernant les pauvres de Rouen,* i, pp. xxviii, 3.

[94] Ibid. La Madeleine traditionally provided for abandoned infants, often sending them to wetnurses in the countryside (see i, pp. xxviii–ix).

[95] *Chronique normande,* 67.

miserable persons infected with the disease of leprosy' would be cared for 'more devotedly and more carefully', and stated that the leprous were to have 'a sufficiency of victuals'.[96] He instructed the archbishop of Rouen to annex the church of Saint-Julien to La Madeleine so that, when the office of rector, priest or administrator became vacant, the prior of La Madeleine or a nominee would take corporal possession of the church, and ensure that divine office was celebrated there, and the sacraments administered, 'as has been the custom there thus far'.[97] Moreover, he ordered that temporal affairs were to be managed in such a way that 'there should not be a lacking of humanity and charity for the miserable persons staying there and who will live there in the future'.[98] He decreed that 'a sufficiency of temporals should be administered to every single one of these persons, so that they should not have to gather timber through need of victuals'.[99]

These provisions may reflect the high status of the women at Salle-aux-Puelles: even if they had not been sick, it would have been inappropriate for them to have had to go out to gather firewood. Above all, however, it is striking that Charles V's charter conveys a compassionate outlook, describing the leprous women as 'miserable persons' who should be treated with humanity. This compassionate tone challenges the view that attitudes towards the leprous became less positive in the fourteenth century, particularly following the Black Death, when fears grew about the spread of disease through miasmatic air.[100] By contrast, here, in 1366, a document issued by the king of France appears to reflect genuine concern about the suffering and needs of the leprous.

It is also clear that, in 1366, it was expected that there would be lepers at Salle-aux-Puelles in the future, and it was believed that they should be provided for according to established customs in the *leprosarium*. In July 1377 Pope Gregory XI (1370–8) confirmed the donation when he instructed the bishop of Paris to annex and unify the church of Saint-Julien and the house of Salle-aux-Puelles to La Madeleine hospital. He also provided for the continuation of spiritual and bodily care at Salle-aux-Puelles, ordering the bishop to ensure 'that in the said church and house there are as many chaplains and ministers as there are now and is the custom, and that in the

---

[96] 'miserabilibus personis morbo lepræ infectis … devotius & curiosius … sufficientiam victualium': appendix 2, no. 13(b) (transcribed from a ?seventeenth-century copy, pp. 1–2).

[97] 'sicut est inibi hactenus consuetum': ibid. (printed copy, p. 2).

[98] 'ne quid in miserabilibus personis inibi morantibus & quæ ibi degent imposterum humanitatis & temporalitatis desit': ibid. (printed copy, p. 2).

[99] 'quinimo unicuique ipsarum personarum ita sufficienter ministretur in temporalibus, quod super victualium penuriâ non habeant materiam conquirendi': ibid. (printed copy, p. 2).

[100] On changing responses to leprosy in the fourteenth century see Brenner, 'Recent perspectives', 390–1, 392.

church divine offices are served, and that the sick in the house are received and nourished as previously'.[101]

Despite its small size, Salle-aux-Puelles was evidently viewed as a significant institution in thirteenth- and fourteenth-century Rouen. Eudes Rigaud visited the *leprosarium* regularly, and drew up detailed statutes. In the fourteenth century, the original royal endowment by Henry II and the community's wealth were still remembered, leading Charles V of France to dispose of it as a gift to La Madeleine hospital. The history of Salle-aux-Puelles sheds an important light on the lives of leprous women in medieval Rouen, and on how their circumstances altered as wider changes occurred in the city.

Small and ephemeral leper houses

As was the case for other major cities, such as Paris, Toulouse and London, there were a number of small *leprosaria* surrounding Rouen.[102] Many of these served villages, and were presumably locally administered. Nonetheless, some were connected to Mont-aux-Malades or to each other, and many had relationships with Rouen parishes. Arrangements were made around 1266 for a leper house to be built at Sotteville-lès-Rouen, south of the river, on land belonging to Mont-aux-Malades. The treasurers of the church of Sotteville paid the nominal sum of 5 *sous* annual rent for the land, which was 'as it were granted in alms'.[103] The arrangement was confirmed by the dean of Saint-Cande-le-Vieux, a collegiate church exempt from the authority of the archbishop of Rouen, which controlled the patronage of Sotteville and four other suburban parish churches.[104] The involvement of the treasurers of Sotteville suggests that the local parish was to oversee the new *leprosarium*. Yet, it was also connected to Mont-aux-Malades, revealing that Rouen's largest leper house potentially had a wider purview than its own resident

---

[101] 'quod in ecclesia et domo predictis sint tot capellani et ministri sicut nunc sunt et esse consueuerunt ac in ecclesia in diuinis deseruiatur et infirmi in dicta domo recipiantur et alimententur sicut prius': appendix 2, no. 29 (quotation from original bull of July 1377). It is not clear why Gregory XI here instructed the bishop of Paris as opposed to the archbishop of Rouen.

[102] For Paris see Dorothy-Louise Mackay, *Les Hôpitaux et la charité à Paris au XIIIe siècle*, Paris 1923, 74–6; for Toulouse see John H. Mundy, 'Hospitals and leprosaries in twelfth- and early thirteenth-century Toulouse', in John H. Mundy, Richard W. Emery and Benjamin N. Nelson (eds), *Essays in medieval life and thought: presented in honor of Austin Patterson Evans*, New York 1955, 181–205; for London see Honeybourne, 'Leper hospitals'.

[103] 'quasi elemosinatam': appendix 2, no. 14.

[104] Ibid; Lemoine and Tanguy, *Rouen*, 36–7; P. Duchemin, *Sotteville-lès-Rouen, et le faubourg de Saint-Sever*, Rouen 1893, repr. Paris 1990, 20–1.

Small and ephemeral leper houses in the environs of Rouen

Location	Dedication	Documentary references	Other information
Bois-Guillaume	Sainte Véronique (Sainte Venisse)	Testament of John Hardi, 1304, ADSM, G7137; testament of Simon de Mara, 1447, ADSM, G3437; register of Rouen cathedral, 1476–9, at 26 Apr. 1479, ADSM, G2140, fo. 199r; Du Plessis, *Description*, ii. 149; Fournée, 'Maladreries', 129–30.	One of the leper houses 'of the four gates of Rouen'. Served Bois-Guillaume, and the Rouen parishes of Saint-Godard and Saint-Laurent. In 1549 a leprous man was residing there.
Darnétal	Saint Claude and Saint Christophe	Testament of John Hardi, 1304, ADSM, G1236, G7137; Du Plessis, *Description*, ii. 149; Fournée, 'Maladreries', 68, 70.	Located near the bridge of Darnétal; served the local parishes of Longpaon and Carville, and the Rouen parishes of Saint-Vivien and Saint-Nicaise.
Moulineaux?	Saint Marc?	Du Plessis mentions the chapel of Saint Marc at Moulineaux, unified to the hospital of Bourg-Achard by 1738: *Description*, ii. 662; Fournée, 'Maladreries', 106.	Existence not certain.
Porte Saint-Ouen, Rouen	Not known	?Eighteenth-century copy of an act of the *bailli* of Rouen, Dec. 1283, BM, Rouen, Tiroir 324, folder 1, fo. 2r; Chéruel, *Histoire*, i. 285–8.	Described as the 'lepers' cabin'.
Répainville	Not known	Testament of John Hardi, 1304, ADSM, G1236, G7137.	

Place	Dedication	Sources	Notes
Saint-Léger-du-Bourg-Denis	Sainte Marguerite	Testament of John Hardi, 1304, ADSM, G1236, G7137; testament of Simon de Mara, 1447, ADSM, G3437; register of Rouen cathedral, 1476–9, at 26 Apr. 1479, ADSM, G2140, fo. 199r; account book of Saint-Maclou parish, Rouen, 1585–6, at 3 Sept. 1586–Christmas 1586, ADSM, G6897, fo. 89r–92v; Du Plessis, *Description*, ii. 149; Fournée, 'Maladreries', 111.	One of the leper houses 'of the four gates of Rouen'. Served the Rouen parishes of Saint-Maclou, Saint-Paul and Saint-Cande-le-Vieux. In ruins in September 1586, when it was rebuilt to accommodate two leprous women.
Saint-Sever	Not known	Testament of John Hardi, 1304, ADSM, G1236, G7137; testament of Simon de Mara, 1447, ADSM, G3437; register of Rouen cathedral, 1476–9, at 26 Apr. 1479, ADSM, G2140, fo. 199r.	One of the leper houses 'of the four gates of Rouen'.
Sotteville-lès-Rouen	Not known	Charter of January 1266, ADSM, 25HP1(16)(ii); Duchemin, *Sotteville-lès-Rouen*, 20–1.	Founded c. 1266 on land belonging to Mont-aux-Malades.
Yonville (Saint-Gervais)	Not known	Testament of John Hardi, 1304, ADSM, G1236, G7137; testament of Simon de Mara, 1447, ADSM, G3437; register of Rouen cathedral, 1476–9, at 26 Apr. 1479, ADSM, G2140, fo. 199r; Du Plessis, *Description*, ii. 149.	One of the leper houses 'of the four gates of Rouen'. Possibly founded by the abbey of Fécamp, which held the patronage of the parish of Saint-Gervais, Rouen. Still standing in the mid-fifteenth century.

community, although it is not known whether Sotteville's leper house was actually constructed.[105]

Four small *leprosaria*, at Yonville or Saint-Gervais (immediately west of Rouen), Saint-Sever (south), Saint-Léger-du-Bourg-Denis (east) and Bois-Guillaume (north), were collectively known in the fourteenth and fifteenth centuries as the leper houses 'of the four gates of Rouen'.[106] While none of these was located in close proximity to a city gate, their locations do mark the four main directions of entry to and exit from Rouen. It is possible that lepers encountered at each of the four principal gates, the Portes Cauchoise, Beauvoisine, de Robec and du Pont, were sent to these *leprosaria*.[107] The leper house at Saint-Léger-du-Bourg-Denis, dedicated to Sainte Marguerite, served the Rouen parishes of Saint-Maclou, Saint-Paul and Saint-Cande-le-Vieux, while the house at Bois-Guillaume, dedicated to Sainte Véronique, catered for lepers from the parishes of Saint-Laurent and Saint-Godard, as well as Bois-Guillaume itself.[108] Much less is known about the *leprosaria* at Yonville and Saint-Sever, but these too may have had relationships with specific Rouen parishes. In April 1479 the lepers of Bois-Guillaume and Saint-Léger-du-Bourg-Denis appealed to the chapter of Rouen cathedral regarding their wish that only the lepers of the four gates should enjoy the cathedral's alms.[109] This suggests that these four *leprosaria* did share a collective identity, and that they were relatively poor establishments, whose residents were among those lepers who received alms at the doors of the cathedral. Indeed, many smaller *leprosaria* depended upon the proceeds of begging.[110] A year earlier, on 14 April 1478, the cathedral chapter had decreed that lepers could not gather at the doors on Sundays and feast days: otherwise, their monthly alms distribution would cease.[111] The testament of John Hardi, issued in 1304, mentions the presence of poor lepers at Rouen on Good Friday and during Ascension, and endowed an alms distribution at the cathedral for lepers.[112] It appears that, in the fourteenth and fifteenth centuries, both itinerant lepers and the sick residing in the smaller *leprosaria* customarily assembled at the cathedral to solicit charity, a practice that was

[105] Bruno Tabuteau (personal communication) suggests that the plans of *c.* 1266 never came to fruition.

[106] 'quatuor ... portarum ... Rothomagen': register of Rouen cathedral, 1476–9, at 26 Apr. 1479, ADSM, G2140, fo. 199r. See also appendix 2, nos 43, 99.

[107] Musset, 'Rouen', 54.

[108] M. Toussaint C. Du Plessis, *Description géographique et historique de la Haute Normandie*, Paris 1740, repr. Brionne 1971, ii. 149; Fournée, 'Maladreries', 111, 129–30.

[109] ADSM, G2140, fo. 199r.

[110] See Rawcliffe, *Leprosy*, 289.

[111] ADSM, G2140, fo. 120r.

[112] Appendix 2, no. 43.

regulated in the late 1470s, perhaps due to concern regarding the unsightliness of lepers and potential risks to public health.[113]

John Hardi's testament also refers to leper communities at Darnétal and Répainville, which were each to receive 5 *sous* after his death.[114] According to Toussaint Du Plessis, the *leprosarium* at Darnétal, east of Rouen, was located near the village's bridge and served the Rouen parishes of Saint-Nicaise and Saint-Vivien, as well as the local parishes of Longpaon and Carville. Its chapel was dedicated to SS Claude and Christopher.[115] Very little is known about the lepers of Répainville, south-east of Rouen, and it is possible that this community was ephemeral and loosely organised, and lacked its own chapel. Another facility for lepers, also perhaps short-lived, was located much closer to the city, on Rouen's north-eastern boundary. In December 1283 the *bailli* of Rouen granted to the commune 'the perch of the lepers' cabin situated at the Porte Saint-Ouen, Rouen, between the wall of the enclosure of the town and the road to Saint-Nicaise, stretching from the pavement up to the wall of Saint-Ouen'.[116] Although this 'cabin' (*bordellum*) was technically outside the city boundary, it was situated at one of the gates, very close to the abbey of Saint-Ouen. This location was a ditch, a marginal area where earth was stored for the use of the dyers and fullers who worked in the cloth industry.[117] 'Bordellum' can also mean 'brothel'; yet, despite the medieval association of leprosy with lasciviousness, it is unlikely that this was a site of prostitution. The word's most probable meaning here is a basic form of accommodation, suggesting that this was a place where lepers leaving the city, or being prevented from entering, were housed temporarily before joining one of the *leprosaria* or embarking on an itinerant existence. It presumably also had no chapel, and thus offered no long-term spiritual or bodily care to the leprous.

The presence of a facility for lepers immediately outside one of the gates of Rouen in the 1280s raises questions about the extent to which leprosy

---

[113] On how leprosy featured in concerns about the spread of disease in Rouen following the Black Death see Elma Brenner, 'Leprosy and public health in late medieval Rouen', in Linda Clark and Carole Rawcliffe (eds), *The fifteenth century*, XII: *Society in an age of plague*, Woodbridge 2013, 123–32, 138.

[114] Appendix 2, no. 43.

[115] Du Plessis, *Description*, ii. 149; Fournée, 'Maladreries', 68, 70.

[116] 'perchiam Bordelli leprosorum sitam ad portam sancti audoeni Rothomagi Inter muram clausturae villae ex una parte et cheminum quo Itur ad sanctum nigasium ex altera sicut se porportat a pavimento usque ad murum sancti audoeni': BM, Rouen, Tiroir 324, folder 1, ? eighteenth-century copy of an act of the *bailli* of Rouen, December 1283, fo. 2r. The full charter of December 1283 is printed in A. Chéruel, *Histoire de Rouen pendant l'époque communale, 1150–1382*, Rouen 1843–4, i. 285–8. This grant and the 'lepers' cabin' are discussed in Brenner, 'The care of the sick and needy', 346.

[117] Gauthiez, 'Urban development', 43, 48.

was a source of fear and anxiety in the city in the thirteenth century.[118] Like the numerous charters in Mont-aux-Malades' archive, the establishment of several smaller *leprosaria* around the city by the fourteenth century undoubtedly reflects the fact that lepers were a key focus of Christian charity. Nonetheless, it also reveals that it was considered necessary to accommodate sufferers at a distance from the city, and to establish institutions that served the sick from villages and suburban areas as well as from Rouen itself. While Salle-aux-Puelles had much in common with Mont-aux-Malades in terms of the royal patronage that it enjoyed, its fine chapel and its provision for high-status residents, the other *leprosaria* were very different in character. This range of institutional forms reflects the multiple social and religious statuses of lepers and, in the case of Salle-aux-Puelles, the distinctions that were made according to gender. Most strikingly, it is clear that relationships with Rouen parishes were fundamental to the foundation and continuing existence of many leper houses. These links provide a broader context for the association of Mont-aux-Malades with twenty-one parishes. Parishes functioned as a conduit for charitable donations to the *leprosaria*, and parishes made arrangements for the care of leprous parishioners until as late as the end of the sixteenth century.[119] The charity of the people of Rouen reflects not only religious practice, but also a sense of responsibility towards those afflicted with leprosy within their immediate social unit, the parish. Yet, while parish involvement sustained a link between the *leprosarium* and the city, it also supported the separation of lepers from mainstream society.

[118] For Archbishop Peter de Collemezzo's rules for Mont-aux-Malades of May 1237, which indicate concern about leprosy and contagion at this early date, see pp. 48–9 above and pp. 99–100 below.

[119] For example, in 1586 the parishioners of Saint-Maclou, Rouen, arranged for two parishioners suspected of having leprosy to be examined and, when confirmed, accommodated at the leper house of Saint-Léger-du-Bourg-Denis: ADSM, G6897, fos 89r–92v (Sept. 1586–Jan. 1587). See pp. 106–7 below.

4

Leprosy and the Medical World of Rouen

While leprosy sufferers were an obvious object of medical attention, the understanding of the disease, and responses to it, changed in Rouen between the twelfth and fifteenth centuries. The Black Death of the mid-fourteenth century undoubtedly had a great impact on the understanding of disease and attitudes towards the sick, including lepers. However, prior to the plague, it is clear that some parties in Rouen were already concerned about leprosy and contagion, while others did not fear to come into frequent contact with the sick. This variation in attitudes and behaviour suggests that this was a disease that provoked particularly complex responses. This chapter places leprosy in the broader context of medical practices and practitioners in medieval Rouen, and examines the bodily care of lepers, diagnosis and ideas about contagion. Physicians were present in the city from the early Middle Ages, and were often members of the ecclesiastical elite, as well as charitable benefactors. From the thirteenth century, lepers received attention from physicians and surgeons within and outside leper houses, particularly as diagnostic examinations became more common. They also benefited from bodily care in terms of the provision of food, shelter and other necessities. In the fifteenth century, anxieties about leprosy and contagion increased markedly, and the disease featured among those threats targeted in measures for the public health of the city.

The practice of medicine in medieval Rouen

The physical care of the sick and the disabled was wide-ranging in the Middle Ages, involving not only interventions by university-educated physicians, but also care administered by surgeons, barbers, midwives, professed religious, lay religious, family members and friends. Measures aimed at ensuring bodily wellbeing, particularly the provision of food, clothing and shelter, three of the biblical works of mercy, formed an essential part of physical care. As well as enabling carers to fulfil Christian works, such measures reflected the 'non-naturals', which were environmental and psychological factors believed to cause health or illness. The six non-naturals consisted of air, sleep, exercise, diet, bodily evacuation and emotional wellbeing. Like the understanding that health resulted from a balance of the four bodily humours (blood, yellow bile, black bile and phlegm), and that each individual had his or her own specific humoral (complexional) balance, the non-naturals formed part of the Galenic model of health and disease.[1]

The care of the sick ranged from the regulation of the diet and the administration of pharmaceutical substances, to bloodletting and other surgical procedures, to the spiritual care of the soul. Indeed, in medieval thinking, spiritual health was closely linked to bodily health. Canon 22 of the Fourth Lateran Council (1215) instructed physicians to ensure that, before they treated a patient, the individual had first received the care of a priest. This was because 'sickness of the body may sometimes be the result of sin ... when the cause ceases so does the effect'.[2] It was thus believed that it was necessary for the soul to be in good health before the body would recover. Furthermore, a disease in the soul could cause bodily affliction, but medicine to the soul might result in the restoration of the body to good health.[3] This emphasis on the importance of the health of the soul helps to explain both the religious organisation of hospitals and *leprosaria*, and the medical roles fulfilled by many religious men and women.

We know relatively little about medical practices and practitioners in medieval Rouen, especially before the thirteenth century. Although the city had several hospitals and *leprosaria*, and several monasteries, such as the abbeys of Saint-Ouen and Saint-Amand, provided for the sick in their infirmaries, the archives and material remains of these institutions reveal little about medical care. Nonetheless, the names of a small number of early practitioners are known, suggesting that there was a recognisable medical profession in Rouen by at least the eleventh century, possibly centred upon the archbishop's household. Lucien Musset states that there was a significant concentration of medical practitioners in the city, mentioning the physician Durand who witnessed a charter in 1095, the physician Ricoard who had property near the abbey of Saint-Lô in the later twelfth century, and 'Master Osmond the physician', a tenant of the abbot of Préaux in the rue Saint-Amand in 1227.[4]

Several practitioners were present in the city in the thirteenth century. In a charter issued between 1206 and 1218, 'Master Simon, *medicus*, rector of Vatetot' donated a house in the rue Saint-Nicolas, Rouen, to the Augustinian priory of Saint-Lô.[5] Simon's status as 'Master' could indicate that

---

[1]   On the non-naturals see, for example, Luke Demaitre, *Medieval medicine: the art of healing, from head to toe*, Santa Barbara, CA 2013, 23–4.

[2]   'infirmitas corporalis nonnumquam ex peccato proveniat ... cum causa cessante cesset effectus': *Decrees of the ecumenical councils*, i. 245.

[3]   See Peregrine Horden, 'A non-natural environment: medicine without doctors and the medieval European hospital', in Barbara S. Bowers (ed.), *The medieval hospital and medical practice*, Aldershot 2007, 141.

[4]   Musset, 'Rouen au temps des Francs', 72.

[5]   'ego magister Simon medicus persona de Watetot': Léonce de Glanville, *Histoire du prieuré de Saint-Lô de Rouen*, Rouen 1890–1, ii. 376 (no. lv). Musset (p. 72) also mentions

he was formally educated in medicine, although this term was used very flexibly in the Anglo-Norman world, by not only medical practitioners but also secular clergy, craftsmen and others. The word *medicus*, on the other hand, was the widely used term for a medical practitioner in the twelfth and thirteenth centuries.[6] The gift of property in a prime location close to Rouen cathedral indicates that Master Simon was wealthy. Vatetot-sur-Mer was a dependent church of Rouen's La Madeleine hospital, donated by Richard I, king of England.[7] Simon's appointment to this church indicates that he was connected to the community at La Madeleine, and might therefore have played a role in the care of the sick poor, abandoned infants and pregnant women at the hospital. Simon, medical practitioner, also appears as a witness in a charter of about 1210 marking a land grant by a canon of Rouen cathedral, and 'Master Symon, *fisicus*' is listed under the date of 28 March in the cathedral's necrology drawn up in 1329.[8] The term *fisicus* in the latter document is significant, since from the later eleventh century the word *physica* (natural philosophy) denoted medicine based on textual learning, as opposed to *medicina*, which broadly signified the practical art of medicine from the early Middle Ages onwards. By the thirteenth century, medicine was established as a university discipline as part of the broader subject of philosophy, and Simon's description as a *fisicus* could thus suggest that he had received a university education, although he is referred to elsewhere as a *medicus*.[9] He was evidently associated with the cathedral (itself closely linked to La Madeleine), supporting the notion that high-status medical practitioners clustered around the archbishop's household in the thirteenth century.[10] Simon was clearly a member of Rouen's ecclesiastical elite.

Archbishop Eudes Rigaud, who suffered from chronic rheumatism that sometimes rendered him unable to travel for weeks at a time, had at least two physicians in his entourage, Master Maur and Master Peter. While Peter

---

Master Simon in his list of practitioners at Rouen, referring to this charter relating to property in the rue Saint-Nicolas. He appears to date this undated charter to c. 1175, but it was drawn up before John Luce as mayor of Rouen, who was mayor in 1206–7, 1210–12 and 1213–18.

6 Kealey, *Medieval medicus*, 34–5, 39.

7 BM, Rouen, MS Y42, fo. 21v; Dubois, 'Les Rouennais', 29, 149.

8 Ernest Wickersheimer, *Dictionnaire biographique des médecins en France au moyen âge*, Paris 1936, 736 (citing the charter of *c.* 1210 which Simon witnesses); 'Magister Symon fisicus': 'E Rotomagensis ecclesiæ necrologio', in *Recueil des historiens*, xxiii. 361. Wickersheimer lists the Simon who was a witness in about 1210 as a separate individual from the 'Symon' included in the cathedral necrology. However, although the necrology was drawn up in 1329, it lists several individuals from an earlier date (for example, Emma, the vicomtesse [second half of the twelfth century] and Archbishop Eudes Rigaud). Thus, it drew upon an earlier list or book, which almost certainly remembered the Simon, *medicus*, who flourished in the first decades of the thirteenth century.

9 Wallis, *Medieval medicine*, pp. xxi–xxiii.

10 Indeed, Musset describes Simon as a *familier* of the archbishop: 'Rouen', 72.

is described as a *medicus*, Maur is qualified as *fisicus*.[11] The *Register* of Eudes Rigaud also reveals that John Godebout, a monk of Saint-Wandrille, the distinguished Benedictine abbey on the river Seine west of Rouen, was a *medicus*. Although John Godebout was one of five monks residing at the dependent priory of Saint-Saëns in March 1267/8, it is plausible that at some point he served the community of Saint-Wandrille itself.[12] In May 1222 the election of a predecessor of Eudes Rigaud as archbishop, Theobald of Amiens (1222–9), was challenged when a rumour circulated that Theobald was leprous. Pope Honorius III sent three judges delegate, Gervase, bishop of Sées, the dean of Amiens and the archdeacon of Rheims, to inquire carefully into the issue, 'having called faithful *medici* skilled in this matter'.[13] It is not clear whether the pope was instructing a formal medical examination, or whether he expected the physicians merely to advise on the man's reported symptoms. If an examination of the archbishop-elect did take place at Rouen, it would mark a very early instance in Europe of the *iudicium leprosorum*, the procedure by which suspected lepers were examined and diagnosed. Furthermore, the physicians recruited were expected already to be experienced in such matters.[14] Such an examination would also provide further evidence for the presence of practitioners in the city in the thirteenth century, practising within the archiepiscopal milieu.

It is likely that many of the physicians who were active in Rouen between 1100 and 1500 had been educated in Paris. Although there is no firm evidence for the existence of the medical faculty in the University of Paris until the mid-thirteenth century, the city was a centre of medical education from at least the late twelfth century. While Paris could not compete with medical learning at Montpellier and Salerno, it had a number of schools where medical students gathered around a master. Although these masters did not participate in the formation of the university in the early 1200s, by

---

[11] 'magistro Mauro, fisico'; 'magistro Petro, medico nostro': *Regestrum*, 159, 439; *Register*, 174–5, 499 (Master Maur mentioned at 30 May 1253; Master Peter mentioned at 18 August 1262); Victoria Turner, 'Monastic medicine in the visitation records of Eudes Rigaud, archbishop of Rouen (1248–75)', unpubl. BA diss. Cambridge 2009, 2; Davis, *Holy bureaucrat*, 43–4, 79, 80, 160–1.

[12] *Regestrum*, 597–98; *Register*, 687. In March 1267/8 the prior of Saint-Saëns 'was sick' ('infirmabatur'): perhaps John Godebout was there for this reason.

[13] 'advocatis medicis fidelibus, et in hoc peritis': *Honorii III Romani pontificis opera omnia*, ed. C. Horoy, Paris 1879–80, iv, epistolae lib. vi, col. 151 (no. 177). In another letter, dated 18 May 1222, Pope Honorius instructed these three churchmen to examine Theobald's election and to establish that he was a suitable person to be made archbishop: ibid. cols 150–1 (no. 176). See Tabbagh, *Fasti*, 80–1; Peltzer, *Canon law*, 84–6. Theobald was found to be free from leprosy, and he was formally consecrated on 4 September 1222.

[14] The earliest instance of the *iudicium leprosorum* that Luke Demaitre has found involving physicians is an examination which took place in Siena (Italy) in 1250, when a certain Pierzivallus was judged to be leprous by four physicians: *Leprosy*, 37, 65.

the early 1270s they drew up statutes for their faculty, by this time a firm constituent part of the university.[15]

Among the 260 Parisian scholars of medicine whose origins can be traced in the period 1250–1400, twenty-six (that is, 10 per cent) came from the diocese of Rouen, the largest number for any French diocese, reflecting Rouen's proximity to Paris.[16] It is likely that at least some of these scholars returned to their 'home' diocese, and may well have practised in the city of Rouen, where the wealthy burgess population represented a lucrative market. Certainly, Rouen physicians who had studied in Paris are known from the later Middle Ages, by which time the University of Caen, founded in 1432 by King Henry VI of England, also offered medical education.[17] William Desjardins, canon of Rouen cathedral (1421–38), became a master of medicine in Paris in 1408 and served as a regent of medicine there until 1418. From that year if not before, he was resident in Rouen.[18] Desjardins was among the advisors or 'assessors' who participated in the trial of Joan of Arc at Rouen between 9 January and 30 May 1431, and is described in the Latin account of the trial as both a 'doctor of medicine' and a canon of the cathedral. Other doctors of medicine, such as Jean Tiphaine, Roland l'Écrivain and Gilles Quenivet, as well as licenciates of medicine such as Guillaume de la Chambre, were also present at the trial, alongside leading ecclesiastics and doctors of theology and canon law.[19] Their involvement testifies to the high status and influence of men of medical learning in late medieval Rouen, and to the social networks produced by the University of Paris, where Bishop Pierre Cauchon, who oversaw the trial, had studied canon law.[20]

Although Rouen's *medici* in the thirteenth century no doubt had wealthy, high-status clients, such as Eudes Rigaud, they may also have visited the sick in hospitals, *leprosaria* and monastic infirmaries. Eudes Rigaud himself encouraged the presence of practitioners within monastic communities.[21] At the Rouen abbey of La Trinité-du-Mont on 17 May 1262, the archbishop specifically instructed that a physician should be found for the sick and a suitable servant for the infirmary.[22] Surgeons also practised within both

---

[15] Cornelius O'Boyle, *The art of medicine: medical teaching at the University of Paris, 1250–1400*, Leiden 1998, 9–20.

[16] Ibid. 37, 39–40.

[17] On the medical faculty at Caen, for which revised statutes were drawn up in December 1473, see Lyse Roy, *L'Université de Caen aux XVe et XVIe siècles: identité et représentation*, Leiden 2006, 85–95.

[18] Tabbagh, *Fasti*, 200 (no. 144); Wickersheimer, *Dictionnaire biographique*, 239.

[19] *The trial of Joan of Arc*, trans. and intro. Daniel Hobbins, Cambridge, MA 2005, 52, 63, 77, 119, 123, 170, 198.

[20] The faculties of the University of Paris were also directly involved with the trial itself: ibid. 3, 4.

[21] Davis, *Holy bureaucrat*, 80.

[22] *Regestrum*, 429–30; *Register*, 489; Davis, *Holy bureaucrat*, 213 n. 126.

monastic houses and the wider community. These practitioners were clearly distinguished from physicians, since the latter did not intervene manually to treat patients. As is the case for physicians, it is difficult to identify surgeons and their activities before the thirteenth century. The first of a series of miracle stories associated with St Dominic at Rouen between 1261 and 1270 takes place in the parish of Saint-Éloi in 1261, and mentions the unsuccessful intervention of 'a certain surgeon'.[23] A small boy roughly one year old had a wooden spindle whorl stuck in his throat. 'Having tried all the diligence of his art', the surgeon said that the only remedy left was to cut open the child's throat, at which the boy's mother 'fled as if mad'.[24] The child's grandmother then appealed to St Dominic for help, and the boy was carried to the Dominican church and placed at the altar while the brothers were beginning to celebrate mass. When close to death, the child suddenly recovered, vomiting the bloodied whorl into the hands of one of the brothers.[25] As well as reflecting the customary appearance of medical practitioners in miracle tales to demonstrate the futility of medicine in comparison to a saint's healing power, this account suggests that surgeons were a recognisable presence in thirteenth-century Rouen, and were perceived to be highly skilled: this man made use of his 'art'. It is also noteworthy that, in the story, the surgeon was willing to intervene in an emergency situation for which he would probably have received no payment. At least some medical practitioners may have undertaken work on a charitable basis in addition to their paid duties, and they may have been expected to intervene in emergencies of this kind.

Although Rouen's surgeons did not receive a royal statute until that issued by Charles VII in 1453, municipal registers from the later fourteenth century reveal the names of three surgeons, and suggest that at least one of them was charged with visiting the sick in La Madeleine hospital and undertaking other civic duties.[26] A further entry in the registers mentions the activity of an unnamed surgeon. The registers record the *hanses*, municipal welfare contributions distributed to the needy from at least the 1390s, and probably much earlier. This term originated in the *lettres de hanse* that foreign merchants had to purchase to do business in Rouen: the money that they

---

[23] 'quidam chirurgicus': 'Miracula, quae Rothomagi in Normannia ab anno Christi MCCLXI usque ad annum MCCLXX contigerunt', in *Acta Sanctorum Augusti*, i, Antwerp 1733, repr. Brussels 1970, 648. On these miracle stories see Mathilde Cordonnier, 'L'Église, les fidèles et la mort, à travers des miracles de Saint Dominique (Rouen, 1261–1270)', *Tabularia 'Études'* viii (2008), 45–57.

[24] 'qui omnem suae artis expertus industriam ... mater eius quasi amens aufugit': 'Miracula, quae Rothomagi ... contigerunt', 648.

[25] Ibid.

[26] For Charles VII's statute for the surgeons of Rouen, April 1453, see Hue, *La Communauté des chirurgiens*, 26–32.

paid was put towards these welfare distributions.[27] The recipient of a *hanse* from Rouen's civic government on 22 June 1398, Colin Osmont, known as "'le prestre des cays'", was sick and 'in the hands of a surgeon'.[28] On 20 October 1389 an exemption from tax payment was granted 'to Robert de Candos, surgeon, as master surgeon in the city, for visiting the sick of La Madeleine or otherwise, considering his small revenue'.[29] On 14 December 1391 tax deductions were granted to Master Jean Lefebvre, Raoul de Caletot and Robert de Candos, surgeons.[30] Although these grants might appear to indicate the poverty of these men, *hanses* were often granted to individuals connected to the civic government, and Robert de Candos definitely had a civic role, as a 'master surgeon' of the city.[31] The 'small revenue' of Robert de Candos probably referred to the modest amount that he was paid for his duties at the hospital, rather than to the size of his overall income. Nonetheless, surgeons may well have been less wealthy than physicians.

Charles VII's statute for Rouen's surgeons, issued after he had regained control of Normandy at the end of the Hundred Years' War, reveals that the surgeons had a clear professional identity by the mid-fifteenth century, and were anxious to curb illicit practice by empirical practitioners. The document states that prospective surgeons must be examined by the master surgeons and, once authorised to practise, must join the profession's religious confraternity of SS Cosmas, Damian and Lambert, based in the Carmelite church. Charlatans and street entertainers who performed surgical procedures were forbidden from doing so unless they had official permission and practised in the presence of authorised surgeons. The statute also mentions the barbers, who acted as phlebotomists, and the apothecaries, confirming the diversity of surgical and medical activities in the city at this time.[32]

As the city's principal hospital for the sick poor, La Madeleine was an important focus of medical activity in medieval Rouen. Although visiting surgeons such as Robert de Candos, and presumably also visiting physicians, were involved in the care of the sick at La Madeleine, the resident lay sisters fulfilled day-to-day duties, reflecting the key role of women in the care of

---

[27] *Documents concernant les pauvres de Rouen*, i, pp. xxxiv–xxxvi.

[28] 'en mains de cirurgien': ADSM, Archives de la Ville, déliberations, registre A4, fo. 69r; *Documents concernant les pauvres de Rouen*, i, pp. xxxvii, 4–5.

[29] 'à Robert de Candos, surgien, comme maitre surgien en la ville pour visiter les malades de la Madeleine ou autrement, considéré sa petite chevance': Hue, *Communauté des chirurgiens*, 9. For Robert de Candos see Wickersheimer, *Dictionnaire biographique*, 709.

[30] Hue, *Communauté des chirurgiens*, 9. For Jean Lefebvre and Raoul de Caletot see Wickersheimer, *Dictionnaire biographique*, 433, 683.

[31] Hue suggests that these grants indicate the low pay received by the surgeons: *Communauté des chirurgiens*, 9. Panel, however, notes that *hanses* were often granted to individuals employed by the municipality: *Documents concernant les pauvres de Rouen*, i, p. xxxv.

[32] Hue, *Communauté des chirurgiens*, 27–30.

the sick in medieval Western Europe. Women's attention to the sick formed part of their broader preoccupation with physical, domestic activities such as caring for children, preparing food, attending women in childbirth and laying out the dead. As Carole Hill argues, 'Women's domain, as officially endorsed by the Church and understood by custom, was service to the body.'[33]

The lay women at La Madeleine came from relatively affluent back-grounds: they provided a dowry upon entry to the hospital community, usually consisting of a property rent.[34] Among them, certain women took on specialised roles in the hospital. The nurse oversaw the sick ward, assisted by two chambermaids. The woman responsible for beds and bedding received the poor when they arrived at the hospital, taking their clothes and giving them sheets and covers. The pittancer and the cellarer were charged with distributing food to the poor. The midwife cared for women giving birth and abandoned infants received at the hospital, who were fed by four wetnurses.[35] La Madeleine's fifteenth-century memorial book records the name of one such midwife, Agnes La Gorelle, whose name was entered in the obituary in about 1460 or earlier. She 'was the midwife of this house for the space of twenty-five years and held herself charitably towards both the community and the poor'.[36] Among the 757 individuals named in the memorial book are a large number of lay sisters, testifying to their important, valued presence in the hospital community. Arguably their engagement in medical duties, some of which were highly specialised, enabled these women to practise a profession, as well as to fulfil a religious vocation and the Christian duty of charity.

As indicated by the 1453 statute for Rouen's surgeons, there must also have been many 'ordinary practitioners' in the city by the later Middle Ages: surgeons, barbers, apothecaries and midwives who were not formally educated in medicine, but supplied many medical services and treatments to the urban population.[37] In England these practitioners often practised another trade, such as brewing, the wool trade or metalworking.[38] On 28 April 1390 Rouen's municipal government granted an *hanse* of 60 *sous* to the daughter of Martin

---

[33] Carole Hill, *Women and religion in late medieval Norwich*, Woodbridge 2010, 3–4, 134. On women as nurses see Monica H. Green, *Making women's medicine masculine: the rise of male authority in pre-modern gynaecology*, Oxford 2008, 125–6.

[34] Rousseau, 'L'Assistance charitable', i. 61.

[35] Ibid. i. 61–2.

[36] 'que fuit obstetrix istius domus per spacium xxv annorum et utrique conuentui ac pauperibus caritatiue se habuit': BM, Rouen, MS Y42, fo. 6r; Dubois, 'Les Rouennais', 42; Rousseau, 'L'Assistance charitable', i. 62.

[37] Faye Getz coins the term 'ordinary practitioner' or 'independent medical tradesperson', noting that 'it is this person about whom the least is known': *Medicine in the English Middle Ages*, Princeton, NJ 1998, 7.

[38] Ibid. 8.

Fouetel, barber, 'to help her to marry'.[39] It would appear that this barber was in financial need. Barbers engaged in a range of activities, from haircutting and shaving to bloodletting, tooth-drawing and minor surgery.[40]

Apothecaries, who traded in medicinal remedies such as potions, spices and unguents, were also present in Rouen by the thirteenth century.[41] The record of Eudes Rigaud's visit to the abbey of Saint-Ouen on 13 December 1258 states that 'Merchants and apothecaries often came there, and entered the cloister, bringing with them items to sell to the monks there.'[42] The archbishop forbade this practice, which involved lay people infiltrating the cloister; yet reference to it suggests that there was a ready market for the wares of apothecaries among the abbey's monks. Apothecaries sometimes worked in conjunction with physicians: at Westminster Abbey, London, in the mid-fourteenth century, a physician and an apothecary met with the infirmarer once a year to settle financial matters.[43] At Saint-Ouen, a similarly high-status monastery, apothecaries could have been closely involved with the affairs of the infirmary, although the situation described in Eudes Rigaud's *Register* indicates that the monastic community as a whole, not just the infirmary staff, was interested in the products offered by apothecaries.

The bodily care of Rouen's lepers

Although it was recognised in the Middle Ages that advanced cases of leprosy could not be cured, a number of different treatments were administered to the leprous, ranging from measures aimed at preventing the disease from taking root in those who were exhibiting early signs, to palliative therapies to lessen the suffering of those in whom it was fully established.[44] The tending of the bodies of lepers is depicted in medieval art, as part of the iconography of the pious works of saints. St Elizabeth of Hungary is a particularly common subject, depicted bathing lepers. Later medieval artworks, in

[39] 'pour la aidier a marier': ADSM, Archives de la Ville, délibérations, registre A1, fo. 121r; *Documents concernant les pauvres de Rouen*, i. 3. See also Wickersheimer, *Dictionnaire biographique*, 541.

[40] Getz, *Medicine*, 8; Carole Rawcliffe, *Medicine & society in later medieval England*, Stroud 1995, 133.

[41] Rawcliffe, *Medicine & society*, 149.

[42] 'Mercerii et apotecarii aliquotiens veniebant, et ingrediebantur claustrum, secum ibidem afferentes res quasdam monachis vendendas': *Regestrum*, 326; *Register*, 373.

[43] Barbara Harvey, *Living and dying in England, 1100–1540: the monastic experience*, Oxford 1993, 83–4; Rawcliffe, *Medicine & society*, 149–50.

[44] On treatment of leprosy in its early stages see Rawcliffe, *Leprosy*, 207–8.

particular, vividly depict the symptoms as well as the treatment of sufferers from leprosy.[45]

Practitioners

Physicians and surgeons charged high fees, meaning that only certain leprous individuals had access to their care. A leprous countess, for example, was treated by the Montpellier physician Bernard de Gordon (fl. 1283–1308).[46] Practitioners underlined the urgent need to treat leprosy in its early stages, before it had reached the vital organs. Treatments of leprosy, in both its initial and more advanced stages, included regulation of the diet, bathing, the administration of purges to force out bad humours, the application of ointments and poultices to treat ulcers, herbal remedies, bloodletting and cauterisation.[47] Practitioners were sensitive to the environmental conditions in which individual patients lived, and the individual's specific complexional balance. Patients were expected to pay attention themselves to the healthy regulation of the environmental and emotional factors (the Galenic non-naturals) that affected their bodies. Practitioners tended to be reluctant to treat advanced cases of leprosy because the death of the patient would affect their professional status, as well as result in a loss of income.[48] Indeed, it would appear that physicians and surgeons avoided practising in leprosaria, institutions which may not have been able or willing to pay their high fees, and whose sick residents had no hope of recovery. Danielle Jacquart found evidence of only eight physicians and one surgeon working within leprosaria in twelfth- to fifteenth-century France, in contrast to 132 practitioners who examined and diagnosed suspected lepers in other settings.[49]

Occasionally, physicians do appear in connection with leper houses; however, they may well have served as administrators or patrons, rather than playing a medical role.[50] The first master and possible founder of the leper house of St James's at Thanington outside Canterbury was the physician Master Feramin, who was also part of the archiepiscopal household.[51] The earliest known reference to a medical practitioner associated with a hospital or leprosarium in France is found in a charter of 1151, in which the medicus Aubert is said to be 'then looking after the affairs of the lepers' of the leper

---

[45] Christine M. Boeckl, Images of leprosy: disease, religion, and politics in European art, Kirksville, Mo 2011, 59–62.

[46] See. ch. 3 n. 18 above, and Demaitre, Leprosy, 21, 172–3.

[47] Rawcliffe, Leprosy, 205–11, 232–8; Boeckl, Images of leprosy, 59, 60.

[48] Rawcliffe, Leprosy, 208, 210–11.

[49] Danielle Jacquart, Le Milieu médical en France du XIIe au XVe siècle, Geneva 1981, 128.

[50] On physicians as administrators of hospitals, thus furthering the ecclesiastical careers that many of them pursued, see ibid. 130–1.

[51] Sweetinburgh, Role of the hospital, 80.

house of Les Deux-Eaux near Troyes.[52] Another physician, Perrinet, made a donation to the leper house of Troyes in 1269.[53] Feramin and Aubert may well have merely administered the *leprosaria* with which they were linked, while Perrinet was probably no more than a benefactor.

Despite the lack of evidence for the presence of practitioners, the sick residents of Rouen's *leprosaria* clearly benefited from bodily care. The non-leprous lay women resident at Mont-aux-Malades and Salle-aux-Puelles must have played an important nursing role. In the middle decades of the thirteenth century, there were many more lay women than lay men at Mont-aux-Malades: in April 1264, sixteen lay sisters lived alongside five lay brothers.[54] The high-status leprous women at Salle-aux-Puelles were served by maids, who could well have acted as nurses.[55] The palliative treatments that lay women would have administered, such as dietary regulation and the application of ointments and dressings, would have helped to alleviate suffering. The fact that Eudes Rigaud's statutes for Salle-aux-Puelles (August 1249) refer to 'the more sick' and 'the more gravely ill' among the leprous sisters suggests that contemporaries were well aware of the different degrees of severity of the disease, and that palliative care was adjusted accordingly.[56]

Bloodletting

Bleeding was practised at Salle-aux-Puelles and some other *leprosaria*. In his statutes for the female leper house, Archbishop Rigaud ordered that 'The sisters should be bled at their times, if it pleases them, and they should have a competent female bloodletter.'[57] He also instructed that 'For those who are more sick, and those who have been bled outside the community, the prior should provide according to their need.'[58] The statutes of the mixed *leprosarium* of Saint-Ladre at Les Andelys, drawn up before 1380, state that every month each sick person should receive two pots of wine 'for his or her bleeding'.[59] In the 1330s, at the leper house of Saint-Lazare outside Montpellier, a city which housed the leading centre of medical learning in France, the lepers were being bled four times per year by a surgeon remunerated by the

---

[52] 'tunc providens rebus leprosorum': Wickersheimer, *Dictionnaire biographique*, 54; Jacquart, *Milieu médical*, 128; Demaitre, *Leprosy*, 241.

[53] Wickersheimer, *Dictionnaire biographique*, 596.

[54] *Regestrum*, 513; *Register*, 585.

[55] *Regestrum*, 538; *Register*, 615.

[56] 'Infirmioribus', 'gravioribus': *Regestrum*, 101, 102; *Register*, 116, 117.

[57] 'Sorores suis temporibus minuant, sibi si placet, et minutricem habeant competentem': *Regestrum*, 102; *Register*, 117.

[58] 'Infirmioribus autem et minutis extra conventum, prior provideat prout necessitati earum': *Regestrum*, 101; *Register*, 116.

[59] 'pour sa saingnée': *Statuts d'Hôtels-Dieu*, 250.

civic government.[60] Bloodletting was an important feature of both medical practice and monastic life in the Middle Ages. In the strictly medical sense it was believed to act as a prophylactic to maintain the proper bodily balance in those who were prone to an imbalance of the humours. In the monastic context it was practised at regular intervals in the liturgical calendar, to prevent physical and spiritual ill health, diminish sexual urges and provide an opportunity for temporary respite from the usual monastic routine.[61]

Given that bleeding involved a period of recovery, and was thus recognised to cause weakness, the letting of blood from lepers may appear counter-intuitive to modern-day eyes. Admittedly, since Eudes Rigaud's statutes mark a set of theoretical instructions and do not refer explicitly to the sisters bled as being leprous, he may have envisaged this as a procedure only to be carried out on healthy members of the community.[62] However, in medieval medical thinking, it was understood that the accumulation or corruption of blood was an important cause of leprosy, making it logical for phlebotomy to be used as a treatment, at least in the disease's early stages.[63] Nonetheless, it was believed that in advanced cases bleeding would only weaken the sufferer. This related to the belief that leprosy spread from the veins into the flesh: once it was well-established in the flesh, it would not be expunged through the removal of blood from the veins. Yet phlebotomy was still practised in certain instances: to alleviate the breathing problems of very sick lepers and on leprous women who were no longer menstruating.[64]

The statutes for Salle-aux-Puelles indicate that here bloodletting certainly reflected monastic practice; yet it may also have formed part of the physical treatment of leprosy. The phrase 'their times' may well refer to the religious calendar: it was common for monastic bloodletting to take place four times a year, although at Saint-Ladre of Les Andelys it was, in theory, practised once a month.[65] Alternatively, 'their times' could indicate a rota by which

---

[60] Geneviève Dumas, 'Bien public et pratiques de la santé à Montpellier au XVe siècle', in *Actes du colloque Montpellier au moyen âge: bilan et approches nouvelles, les 14 et 15 novembre 2013, Université Montpellier 3*, forthcoming. I thank Dr Dumas for sharing this article with me prior to publication.

[61] Mary K. K. H. Yearl, 'The time of bloodletting', unpubl. PhD diss. Yale 2005, abstract, 1–5, 94–5, and 'Medieval monastic customaries on *minuti* and *infirmi*', in Bowers, *The medieval hospital*, 176–7.

[62] Indeed, in general it was believed that bloodletting should only be performed on the healthy members of a religious community, to minimise the disruption to community life: idem, 'Time of bloodletting', 85.

[63] Demaitre, *Leprosy*, 260–1; Rawcliffe, *Leprosy*, 233.

[64] Rawcliffe, *Leprosy*, 232–4.

[65] For the Cistercians, these times were February, April, a date close to the feast of St John the Baptist (24 June), and September; the times may have been similar at Salle-aux-Puelles, at which the order followed is not known: Yearl, 'Time of bloodletting', 88, 94; Green, *Making women's medicine masculine*, 122, 124. For Les Andelys see *Statuts d'Hôtels-Dieu*, 250.

small groups of women were bled in rotation.[66] The specification for a female bloodletter (*minutrix*) to be used not only indicates that female medical practitioners were active in thirteenth-century Rouen, but also reflects widely-held beliefs that religious women should be protected, as far as possible, from contact with men from outside the cloister. This necessitated the supply of female medical expertise, which could be available externally or within the religious community itself. For example, two nuns at the Dominican house of Longchamp, west of Paris, acted as barber-surgeons in the fourteenth and fifteenth centuries.[67] It was still recognised that, in serious situations, male medical practitioners should be brought into the cloister.[68]

It appears that bloodletting could take place outside Salle-aux-Puelles itself: thus, the women (leprous or not) did leave the cloister for this purpose.[69] Bleeding was also voluntary. Those who had been bled were put in the same category as the 'more sick', suggesting that the physical impact of phlebotomy was appreciated, as was also the case at Les Andelys, where those who had been bled replenished their fluids by drinking wine.[70] Sisters who had been bled at Salle-aux-Puelles probably spent a period of time in the *leprosarium*'s infirmary, a building mentioned in the record of Eudes Rigaud's visit on 9 December 1258.[71]

Diet

It was also believed that the proper humoral balance within the body could be restored through dietary regulation. Lepers were encouraged to consume foodstuffs that were mild and moist, such as eggs, poultry, fresh fish, freshly baked bread, good pork and light wine.[72] Carole Rawcliffe notes that many *leprosaria* were well equipped to provide such a diet: they kept pigs, hens and cattle, and some had the right to fish in nearby rivers.[73] Mont-aux-Malades certainly had a rich supply of herrings through the gifts of Henry II, although these may have been salted rather than fresh.[74] Food and drink also had great religious significance. The eucharist represented the consumption of

---

[66] See Yearl, 'Medieval monastic customaries', 178.

[67] Green, *Making*, 120–5; Wickersheimer, *Dictionnaire biographique*, 505 (Jeanne de Crespi, d. 1349), 532 (Macée de Chaulmont, d. 22 Mar. 1485).

[68] Green, *Making women's medicine masculine*, 124.

[69] Yearl states that bleeding took place 'in the infirmary, warming room or some other place appointed for the event', i.e., inside the monastery: 'Medieval monastic customaries', 184.

[70] *Statuts d'Hôtels-Dieu*, 250.

[71] *Regestrum*, 325; *Register*, 371–2.

[72] Rawcliffe, *Leprosy*, 213.

[73] Ibid. 214.

[74] Appendix 2, nos 30(e), 30(g).

the body and blood of Christ, and communal eating promoted harmony and sociability in monastic institutions, including *leprosaria*.[75]

Eudes Rigaud's statutes for Salle-aux-Puelles state that the leprous sisters were to have wine, beer and bread daily, fresh meat in the proper season, fish once a week at other times, and five eggs or three herrings on days when they did not eat meat or other fish. These foodstuffs were among those that were considered mild, moist and beneficial to the leprous. However, other tenets in these statutes suggest that the archbishop's dietary provisions did not take specific account of the leprous condition of the sisters at Salle-aux-Puelles. He instructed that the non-leprous clerics and the sisters should share exactly the same food, unless a change needed to be made for a reason such as the offering of hospitality to guests. Furthermore, he ordered abstinence from meat during Lent and solemn feasts.[76] This suggests that, in his provisions for diet as perhaps also in his instructions for bloodletting, the archbishop was establishing ideal monastic practice at Salle-aux-Puelles, rather than instituting special arrangements for lepers.

Dietary provisions made for leprous religious from Rouen's other monastic houses residing at Mont-aux-Malades suggest that here, too, diet did not relate specifically to an individual's physical condition. In the thirteenth century, special arrangements were made for the upkeep of leprous religious from La Madeleine hospital and the abbey of Saint-Ouen residing at Mont-aux-Malades. On the Monday after the feast of St Remigius, October 1261, the prior of La Madeleine confirmed the dietary provision for a leprous brother, Canon Roger, and a leprous sister, Haisia, who had entered Mont-aux-Malades the previous day. Canon Roger was to have the same entitlement to food and drink as a brother (presumably a canon) of Mont-aux-Malades, while Sister Haisia was entitled to the same victuals as a sister.[77] The prior of La Madeleine thus ensured that the two members of his community would be well provided for at Mont-aux-Malades. It would appear that the non-leprous religious at the *leprosarium* had a different diet from the leprous, and that, by virtue of their high religious status, the leprous canon and sister from La Madeleine enjoyed this diet rather than that of their fellow lepers. The diet of the non-leprous may have been perceived to be superior or more enjoyable; alternatively, the significant factor was that the leprous religious from La Madeleine would eat with religious of similar status to themselves.

Special dietary arrangements were also made for leprous monks from the abbey of Saint-Ouen at Mont-aux-Malades. A charter issued by the *leprosarium*'s prior, probably Richard (prior until 1298), on 18 February 1297, established that a monk from Saint-Ouen was to receive bread and wine daily paid for by the abbey, and to have a diet of meat, eggs and herrings. He

[75] Bynum, *Holy feast and holy fast*, 1–2, 3.

[76] *Regestrum*, 101; *Register*, 116.

[77] Appendix 2, no. 32. See p. 54 above.

was to enjoy a pittance of food or drink whenever the canons of Mont-aux-Malades did, as if he were one of them.[78] Once again, leprous religious from another monastic house were aligned with the healthy religious of Mont-aux-Malades, rather than with the lepers. These two examples reveal that not all the resident lepers ate the same diet, and indicate that the specific diet of individual lepers related more to their religious status than to ideas about dietary care. Nonetheless, it is notable that here, again, mild and moist foodstuffs were prescribed for lepers.

Shelter and clothing

Providing lepers with appropriate clothing and warm, dry accommodation also constituted an important part of their bodily care. In his charter of the 1180s in favour of Salle-aux-Puelles, Henry II granted an annual sum of money for the women's sustenance and clothing. He also accorded them the right to take wood from the nearby forest of Rouvray to heat and repair their houses.[79] In the fourteenth century and probably earlier, Mont-aux-Malades had the right to collect wood to burn for its house *La Maladrerie* in the forest of Lyons, where it had received land from Henry II.[80] Given its name, *La Maladrerie* could have been a satellite leper house, although no information survives to confirm this hypothesis. *Leprosaria* in England similarly had rights to wood, kindling, peat and turf. St James's, Bridgnorth, situated just outside royal forests, received dead trees and a daily quantity of kindling from King Henry III; St Nicholas's, Harbledown, itself owned a large amount of wood-land.[81] Wood provided fuel for cooking, heating and brewing, and was also an essential building material.[82]

Clothing was another important means of ensuring that lepers stayed warm; it also signified their social and religious status. Eudes Rigaud's statutes for Salle-aux-Puelles contain detailed provisions regarding clothing, which relate to the leprous sisters' religious identity, high social status and physical condition. The archbishop instructed that the women should all wear the same uniform, a russet coat. They were to receive a tunic and super-tunic every year. They were also to have fur-lined cloaks 'according to their need', shoes, and linen blouses and sheets:[83]

---

[78] Ibid. no. 86; Langlois, *Histoire*, 124–5. See p. 54 above.

[79] Appendix 2, no. 30(i).

[80] Mont-aux-Malades received 140 acres of land in the forest of Lyons from Henry II in the 1170s: appendix 2, no. 30(e). A charter of Philip VI of France, issued on 15 Feb. 1330, shows that Mont-aux-Malades had appealed to him regarding the infringement of its rights in the forest of Lyons, including the right to collect wood for its house *La Maladrerie*: appendix 2, no. 76(a).

[81] Rawcliffe, *Leprosy*, 331–2.

[82] Ibid.

[83] 'prout necessitati earum'. *Regestrum*, 101–2; *Register*, 116–17.

Item, they should have linen clothes, that is, two blouses and two linen sheets, every year at least, and if more ought to be made for the more gravely sick on account of their needs, they should be made according to the judgement of the prioress. Indeed, the prioress should be discreet, so that she recognises and shows pity towards the infirmities of the sisters, according to the available resources of the house.[84]

Linen was evidently considered an appropriate fabric with which to clothe lepers: it may have been held not to irritate inflamed, ulcerated flesh. In this respect, its provision can be viewed as part of the palliative care of the leprous. The further specification that 'the more gravely sick' should be permitted to have more linen blouses and sheets if necessary also shows awareness of the physical implications of leprosy. As a result of the wounds and sores which afflicted their bodies, the women's sheets and clothing may have quickly became soiled, meaning that fresh linen was required. Medical texts taught that clean clothing and personal cleanliness were important in the treatment of skin diseases.[85] The provision of clean linen was also emphasised elsewhere: the statutes of the Hôtel-Dieu-le-Comte at Troyes, issued on 10 June 1263, specified that sheets were to be washed at least once a week, and once a day if necessary.[86] Clothing at the *leprosarium* at Sherburn, County Durham, was washed twice a week.[87]

The fact that fur-lined cloaks were made available on the basis of need at Salle-aux-Puelles might indicate that only extremely sick women were permitted to wear this very warm clothing. However, fur was also a marker of high status, suggesting that there were reasons other than bodily care for its availability at this *leprosarium* for aristocratic women. When confirming a grant to Mont-aux-Malades in May 1223, Richard Marshal, the future earl of Pembroke (1231–4), symbolically donated a pair of fur gloves in return for a pair of 'single gloves' annually.[88] The russet coat worn by the women may also have reflected their social status, as well as their membership of a religious community that shared a common habit.[89]

The supply of clothing was one of the corporal works of mercy, and linen and woollen clothing was provided at many English *leprosaria*, where a uniform was also required.[90] Like the regulation of the diet and bloodletting,

---

[84] 'Item, vestes lineas habeant, videlicet duas camisias et duo linteamina, omni anno ad minus, et si gravioribus plus oporteat fieri pro sua necessitate, fiat eis iuxta arbitrium priorisse, que adeo sit discreta, quod sciat et velit compati infirmitatibus aliarum, prout domus suppetent facultates': *Regestrum*, 102; *Register*, 116–17.

[85] Rawcliffe, *Leprosy*, 330.

[86] *Statuts d'Hôtels-Dieu*, 116.

[87] Rawcliffe, *Leprosy*, 330.

[88] Appendix 2, no. 85.

[89] Eudes Rigaud's statutes describe the uniform as a 'habitus': *Regestrum*, 101.

[90] Rawcliffe, *Leprosy*, 329–31.

clothing was as much a part of the religious life of the leper house as a form of bodily care. Nonetheless, there were undoubtedly concerted efforts to provide palliative care in Rouen's *leprosaria*, through the provision of food, shelter and clothing, as well as through more interventive measures such as phlebotomy and the treatment of ulcers and sores. Much as the care of the soul was intimately connected to that of the body, palliative care was interwoven with the daily routine and customary monastic practices of the leper house community.

Leprosy and contagion

The almost universal location of *leprosaria* outside medieval towns and cities has often been attributed to fears about contagion. However, François-Olivier Touati has done much to change our thinking on this subject, arguing that leprosy was not associated with contagion until from about 1220–30, and only definitively from the early fourteenth century. The ancient understanding of the disease, upon which medieval thinking was based, saw leprosy as a chronic illness that resulted from internal bodily corruption caused by an imbalance of the humours. Thus, leprosy was not believed to result from the action of external factors upon the body. However, the Latin translation of Arabic medical texts in the eleventh and twelfth centuries, particularly Avicenna's *Canon*, rendered into Latin by Gerard of Cremona before 1187, did introduce ideas concerning contagion. Constantine the African's translation of Haly Abbas's *Pantegni*, a translation completed before about 1098, stated that the disease could be contracted through the inhalation of noxious air (miasma) emanating from sick bodies, and through living and speaking with lepers. Avicenna's *Canon* also referred to corrupt air and close proximity to lepers, as well as to the negative effects of hot air combined with bad food. Nonetheless, both texts begin by outlining the humoral causes of the disease: in Avicenna, the contagious factors are only auxiliary. By the early fourteenth century, the association of miasmatic air with the transmission of disease was firmly established in medical thinking, and several writers, such as Bernard de Gordon and Peter of Abano, argued for the role of corrupt air and physical contact in causing leprosy. However, it was only following the Black Death, a phenomenon attributed to the effects of miasma, that contagion was viewed as the primary cause of leprosy. In 1363 the surgeon Guy de Chauliac (c. 1300–68) listed corrupt air and contact as its principal causes.[91]

In Rouen, concerns about the transmission of leprosy were evidently felt by some parties from at least the thirteenth century. Rules drawn up

---

[91] Touati, 'Contagion',185–98, and 'Historiciser la notion de contagion: l'exemple de la lèpre dans les sociétés médiévales', in Sylvie Bazin-Tacchella, Danielle Quéruel and Évelyne Samama (eds), *Air, miasmes et contagion: les épidémies dans l'antiquité et au moyen âge*, Langres 2001, 175–83.

for Mont-aux-Malades by Peter de Collemezzo in May 1237 suggest that this archbishop believed that leprosy was contagious. The text states that 'If it should happen that the parents or relatives of the lepers or others ... are permitted to sit or drink with the lepers, we will consider them to be infected.'[92] The date of this document corresponds with Touati's chronology for the emergence of ideas about leprosy and contagion. Furthermore, the implied belief that proximity to or contact with the sick was dangerous accords with the Latin translations of the Arabic medical works discussed above. This rare indication in the sources from Rouen of ideas about how leprosy was transmitted could reflect widely-held views. The verb *inficere* ('to infect') was used in relation to leprosy in other contexts in the mid-thirteenth century, but although it appears to reflect its modern-day sense, it may not have had exactly the same meaning in the thirteenth century as today.[93] Certainly, much later, in sixteenth-century Germany, 'infection' remained a very flexible concept.[94] De Collemezzo may, therefore, have believed that those who came into physical proximity or contact with the leprous would be tainted or contaminated in some way (perhaps as much by the diseased state of lepers' souls as by their bodily decay and stench), rather than literally contracting the disease.

Furthermore, the archbishop's statement suggests that, at this time, there was in fact frequent contact between the lepers of Mont-aux-Malades and family members and other people from outside the community. De Collemezzo also referred to gifts from parents and relatives, further indicating that family visits were the norm.[95] Such visits, like the annual fair of Saint-Gilles at Mont-aux-Malades, sustained links between the leper community and mainstream society, and their occurrence implies that many people were not greatly concerned about leprosy and contagion.

Peter de Collemezzo's concerns about contact between the leprous and the non-leprous at Mont-aux-Malades are echoed in a set of synodal statutes from the archdiocese of Rouen, reconfirming earlier precepts and adding new ones, which were attributed to this archbishop in an edition of the eighteenth century. This attribution, however, is problematic: the editor Guillaume Bessin states that the statutes date from no later than 1235, and Peter did not become archbishop until October 1236. However, the new

---

[92] 'si vero contigerit quod aliqui parentes uel consanguinei leprosorum vel alii ... permittantur consedere vel bibere cum leprosis, nos ipsos contingamus Infici': AN, Paris, S4889B, dossier 13, doc. (xxi), fo. 2r.

[93] Touati cites the reference to 'lepram quae inficit ... et lepram quae non inficit' in the *Summa aurea* of Hostiensis composed in 1253: 'Historiciser', 175.

[94] Annemarie Kinzelbach, 'Infection, contagion, and public health in late medieval and early modern German imperial towns', *Journal of the History of Medicine and Allied Sciences* lxi (2006), 373–5.

[95] AN, Paris, S4889B, dossier 13, doc. (xxi), fo. 1r.

set of precepts added to the original statutes was undoubtedly authored by de Collemezzo.[96] Perhaps the version of earlier precepts was drawn up by his predecessor, Archbishop Maurice (1231–5); in any case, these would have been enforced by Peter.[97] The earlier precepts state that lepers are to be prevented from entering cities and castles, and from sitting in taverns and houses to drink.[98] The latter provision is similar to Archbishop Peter's uneasiness about the parents or relatives of lepers sitting or drinking with them. The synodal instructions also indicate an anxiety about contagion, since they aim to keep lepers away from crowded places. They could too reflect concern about the effect that the shocking physical appearance and stench of lepers could have on members of mainstream society. The synodal statutes emphatically restricted the movements and actions of lepers; with regard to leprous individuals who contravened the rules, 'we will not show them justice'.[99]

The precepts also stated that, under pain of excommunication, no one was to give anything to lepers within cities or towns. Equally, however, they instructed priests to compel their parishioners, through the parish dean, 'to provide for lepers'.[100] A clear distinction was made between begging in urban places, which was unacceptable, and the need to supply charity to lepers (presumably, in *leprosaria*), which was an essential Christian duty. These synodal statutes indicate that there was significant concern in Normandy in the first part of the thirteenth century about controlling and regulating the presence of lepers within urban society. Although the leprous had a right, as Christians, to be supported within leper houses, outside these institutions they were understood to pose a threat to public health and to be potentially disruptive of everyday life. Even though Rouen's municipal government was becoming increasingly well-established in this period, the archbishops of Rouen laid down these rules, underlining their key role in civic as well as ecclesiastical matters at this time.

Following the Black Death, the issues of public health and the spread of disease became more pressing. There was increased anxiety about pollution, stench and 'infection', attributed to features of urban life such as pigs, poultry, open latrines, the slaughter of animals outside of abattoirs,

---

96 *Concilia Rotomagensis provinciae*, ed. Guillaume Bessin, Rouen 1717, second section, 52–3.

97 For Archbishop Maurice see Tabbagh, *Fasti*, 82–4.

98 *Concilia Rotomagensis*, second section, 72–3; Bruno Tabuteau, 'Les Léproseries dans la Seine-Maritime du XIIe au XVe siècle', unpubl. MA diss. Rouen 1982, 204.

99 'non exhibemus eis justitiam' and 'non exhibebimus eis justitiam de injuria facta': *Concilia Rotomagensis*, second section, 72–3; Tabuteau, 'Léproseries', 204.

100 'ad providendum leprosis': *Concilia Rotomagensis*, second section, 73; Tabuteau, 'Léproseries', 204.

and contaminated water and food.[101] The 1321 'Lepers' Plot', when lepers and Jews were accused of poisoning the waters of the kingdom of France, reveals that such anxieties pre-dated the arrival of the plague.[102] After the Black Death, Rouen experienced outbreaks of plague throughout the later fourteenth and fifteenth centuries.[103] There were further epidemics in the sixteenth and seventeenth centuries, with what appears to have been the last outbreak in 1668–9.[104]

As in other northern French towns, official measures to combat the spread of disease were enacted in Rouen from the fifteenth century, considerably later than in areas of Europe further south, where northern Italian cities took the lead.[105] A royal ordinance relating to fifteenth-century Rouen testifies to the range of public health concerns at this time, and to the fact that leprosy, although by then becoming less prevalent, featured among these concerns. The ordinance, regulating the activities of butchers selling meat in two new butcheries of the city, in the *halles* of the *Vieux Marché* and at the Porte Beauvoisine, was issued by the *bailli* of Rouen and Gisors on 28 June 1432 and confirmed by Charles VIII (1483–98) in November 1487. It evidences strategies to protect the 'common public good' from disease.[106] The document states that bad meat can be 'of very great danger and prejudice to human creatures'.[107] It aims to ensure that no pork, beef or lamb 'infected with any diseases' is on sale at the butcheries.[108] No butcher is to sell beef infected with 'fy' (believed to be a bovine form of leprosy) or any other

---

[101] On such concerns, and the measures taken to address them, in late medieval England see Carole Rawcliffe, *Urban bodies: communal health in late medieval English towns and cities*, Woodbridge 2013. On these concerns in late medieval Rouen see Philippe Lardin, 'Les Rouennais et la pollution à la fin du moyen âge', in Élisabeth Lalou, Bruno Lepeuple and Jean-Louis Roch (eds), *Des Châteaux et des sources: archéologie et histoire dans la Normandie médiévale: mélanges en l'honneur d'Anne-Marie Flambard Héricher*, Mont-Saint-Aignan 2008, 399–427.

[102] Barber, 'Lepers, Jews and Moslems', 1–17.

[103] Fournée, 'Les Normands face à la peste', 35, 36; Sadourny, 'Des Débuts', 100. For the plague outbreak of 1499 see ADSM, Archives de la Ville, délibérations, registre A9, fo. 318r; Lardin, 'Rouennais', 418.

[104] Fournée, 'Normands', 36.

[105] Neil Murphy, 'Plague ordinances and the management of infectious diseases in northern French towns, c. 1450–c. 1560', in Clark and Rawcliffe, *The fifteenth century*, xii. 139–59, esp. pp. 150–8. Urban responses in England were also much slower than in northern Italy, although decisive measures were taken in a number of localities in the fourteenth and fifteenth centuries: Rawcliffe, *Urban bodies*, 30–5.

[106] 'bien commun de la chose publique': 'Statuts des bouchers vendant dans les halles du Vieux-Marché et de la Porte Beauvoisine, à Rouen', in *Ordonnances des rois de France*, 39–45. On the butcheries at the Porte Beauvoisine and the *Vieux Marché* see Periaux, *Dictionnaire*, 35–6, 61, 147, 658.

[107] 'très-grant dangier et prejudice des creatures humaines': 'Statuts des bouchers', in *Ordonnances des rois de France*, 39.

[108] 'entechiez d'aucunes maladies': ibid. 41.

disease, or infected lamb. The butchers also must not market any 'beast whatever it is that comes from a leper house'.[109]

This document reveals an understanding that animals could become infected with certain diseases, and that the humans who subsequently consumed their meat risked themselves becoming sick. The instruction regarding the meat of animals reared at *leprosaria* is emphatic, encompassing all livestock 'whatever it is'. This indicates that it may have been problematic for leper houses to sell their agricultural produce at this time. By the fifteenth century, when ideas about disease transmission through corrupt air, physical contact and contaminated food and drink circulated increasingly widely, royal authorities were evidently concerned about leprosy and contagion at Rouen, although the attitudes of the wider population are more difficult to gauge.[110]

Diagnosing leprosy

While a number of forms of bodily care were available within leper houses, physicians and surgeons were largely absent from these institutions. The most likely setting in which a leprosy sufferer would have encountered a physician or surgeon was at a diagnostic examination. The legal procedure whereby a person who was suspected of having leprosy was examined, and a judgement was made, was known as the *iudicium leprosorum* ('judgement of lepers'), and took place in many different parts of Western Europe from the early thirteenth century, if not earlier.[111] Although parish priests could be involved in these procedures, from the middle of the thirteenth century civic officials, medical practitioners and the residents and administrators of *leprosaria* were increasingly responsible for diagnosis.[112] The various parties could differ in their findings, especially since physicians deployed a knowledge of medical theory that was not necessarily shared by their lay counterparts.[113] By the fifteenth century physicians and surgeons played the leading role in examinations, as demonstrated by evidence from Montpellier, where Geneviève Dumas has traced seven such procedures between 1493 and 1497, all involving practitioners.[114]

[109] 'beste quelle qu'elle soit qui vienne de maladerie': ibid. 42.

[110] On anxiety about leprosy and contagion exhibited by the authorities in other northern French towns in the fifteenth and sixteenth centuries see Murphy, 'Plague ordinances', 156. For a longer discussion of leprosy and public health issues in Rouen see Brenner, 'Leprosy and public health', 123–38.

[111] On leprosy examinations in one region, the Pas-de-Calais area of northern France, see Bourgeois, *Lépreux et maladreries*, 25–32.

[112] Demaitre, *Leprosy*, 35–41.

[113] See Bourgeois, *Lépreux*, 30–1.

[114] Dumas, 'Bien public', forthcoming.

There is very little information relating to the *iudicium* in Rouen and its surroundings until as late as the sixteenth century; however, there are indications that examinations at least occasionally took place from the thirteenth century onwards. The inquiry into the election of the suspected leper Theobald of Amiens as archbishop of Rouen in 1222 may have involved an examination by *medici*. On 6 September 1268, when visiting the abbey of Le Tréport, in the far north of Normandy on the coast, Eudes Rigaud found that: 'Brother Richard, formerly a prior [of a priory dependent on the abbey], was held suspected of the disease of leprosy: thus, we ordered that he should undergo an examination in the presence of some monks sent with him.'[115] The examination was apparently to be performed outside the abbey itself; yet monks were to accompany Richard, perhaps to verify the outcome on behalf of the community. Although this examination could plausibly have involved medical practitioners, it still had a strong ecclesiastical flavour, being ordered by the archbishop and witnessed by monks.

When Eudes Rigaud had encountered another case of suspected leprosy a few months earlier, he had not ordered an examination, which suggests that the *iudicium* was not a firmly established practice in the archdiocese of Rouen at this time. At the abbey of Bec-Hellouin (south-west of Rouen), on 3 April 1268, he found that Brother Nicholas of Lendy was suspected of having leprosy. However, in this instance, the archbishop merely advised the abbot 'that he should remove the said brother N. [Nicholas] from there', and was informed that the abbot would send him to Saint-Lambert, a dependent priory where there was only one monk.[116] Thus, there was no mention of an examination: it was simply accepted that the man was indeed leprous, or at least that the possibility was great enough for him to be segregated. Saint-Lambert was considered an ideal place 'where there is not the crowding of people, and where he can have the benefit of the air and much mitigation of his infirmity'.[117] This reference to the lack of people at Saint-Lambert may indicate concern about contagion; equally, however, a quiet, peaceful environment may have been considered beneficial to leprosy sufferers. The air was one of the Galenic non-naturals, the factors that were believed to affect health, and it is clear that overall Eudes Rigaud believed that a change of environment would improve Brother Nicholas's condition. His concern was more with the monk's wellbeing than with any threat that he posed to the health of those around him.

Whether or not they were formally diagnosed, some of the sick residents of Rouen's *leprosaria* may not have suffered from the condition now clini-

---

[115] 'Frater Ricardus, quondam prior, suspectus habebatur de morbo lepre, et tunc precepimus ei quod coram aliquibus monachis cum eo missis examinationem subiret': *Regestrum*, 609; *Register*, 701.

[116] 'quod dictum fratrem N. abinde amoveret': *Regestrum*, 623; *Register*, 717.

[117] 'ubi non est frequentia hominum, ubique beneficium aeris et multa infirmitatis sue levimenta habere posset': *Regestrum*, 623; *Register*, 717.

cally known as Hansen's disease. Some individuals plausibly had other skin complaints such as psoriasis and eczema that were mistaken for leprosy. However, excavations of cemeteries associated with *leprosaria* in England and Denmark have found a clear incidence of what would today be viewed as leprosy, suggesting that many cases were correctly diagnosed.[118] These findings are corroborated by the archaeological study of the site of the leper house of Saint-Thomas at Aizier, half-way between Rouen and Le Havre. Archaeologists identified the remains of several individuals showing signs of leprosy, above all in bone changes in the face, particularly in the naso-maxillary area.[119]

Nonetheless, statutes from two French *leprosaria* suggest that those admitted did not always subsequently develop the full symptoms of leprosy. The late twelfth- to mid-thirteenth-century statutes of Saint-Ladre of Noyon, north of Paris, instructed that 'if a burgess is judged to be sick, and it can be found that on the contrary he is not sick, we order that he is put outside the house, and that he is made to pay all his expenses'.[120] The word 'judged' may suggest that a formal examination took place before patients were admitted to the leper house at Noyon. The June 1239 statutes of the *leprosarium* at Lille, issued by Walter, bishop of Tournai, stated that:

> A person who has been received as a leper, and who later cannot be demonstrated to be leprous, should return to where he came from; however, in such a way that, in return for that which he gave at first for his sustenance [an entrance gift], he should be able to return if subsequently he should truthfully be [shown to be] a leper.[121]

This tenet suggests that sometimes there was real uncertainty as to whether the disease was present in a person, particularly in the early stages of his or her symptoms. It also indicates an acceptance that the process of identifying leprosy was neither precise nor infallible. In addition, both sets of statutes point towards the administrative implications of a false admission: to have already paid an entrance gift gave someone who left the community the right to re-enter, while a person who had profited from the goods of the house when not leprous had to repay his or her share. At Rouen, the case of Isabel

---

[118] John Magilton, 'The hospital of St James and St Mary Magdalene, Chichester, and other leper houses', in Bruno Tabuteau (ed.), *Lépreux et sociabilité du moyen âge aux temps modernes*, Rouen 2000, 85; Boldsen, 'Epidemiological approach', 380, 382–3, 384–5.

[119] Niel and Truc, 'La Chapelle Saint-Thomas d'Aizier', 97–101.

[120] 'se un bourgeois est jugiés pour malade et on puet trouver le contraire que il ne soit mie malades, nous commandons que il soit mis hors de le maison et que on li fache paier ses frais de tout que il y aura esté': *Statuts d'Hôtels-Dieu*, 198.

[121] 'qui pro leproso receptus fuerit et postea non esse leprosus convinci poterit redire debet unde venit; ita tamen quod pro pastu suo, quod primo dedit, redire poterit si postea veraciter fuerit leprosus': ibid. 202.

of Avènes at Salle-aux-Puelles, the woman who bore a child and in 1266 asked to leave the *leprosarium*, may mark one instance of misdiagnosis.[122]

By the sixteenth century, leprosy was in decline in Western Europe, but had not yet receded completely. The report of a municipal inspection of Mont-aux-Malades on 19 February 1524 stated that there were three sick individuals there: two men from the parish of Saint-Lô and a woman from the parish of Notre-Dame-de-la-Ronde.[123] Similarly, at the time of the Dissolution of the Monasteries in England in 1539, the leper house of St Giles at Holborn, London, was apparently still providing for up to fourteen sick residents.[124] In the early modern period there was what Luke Demaitre has called 'an increasing elasticity in the identification of leprosy'.[125] This, as well as greater anxiety about the spread of disease in this period of plague, may explain why people continued to be diagnosed with leprosy when it was in fact becoming less and less prevalent. This more flexible definition of leprosy was linked to an increasingly empirical approach which emphasised the signs and description of the disease over the earlier understanding of it based on medical theory and natural philosophy.[126]

Documented cases of leprosy in sixteenth-century Rouen involved examinations, suggesting that by this time the *iudicium leprosorum* was a well-established procedure in the city. These examinations involved both learned medical practitioners and the residents of Rouen's most prominent leper house, but also reflect the administrative oversight of parishes. On 31 October 1536 John du Tremblé, 'suspected of the disease of leprosy', was taken to Mont-aux-Malades, which may have been a key location for such examinations at this time.[127] He was examined by the leprous brothers and sisters, who found that he indeed had leprosy.[128] The official of the parish of Saint-Gervais, Rouen, oversaw the judgement, suggesting that John du Tremblé resided in this parish.[129] It is possible that he was reported by his neighbours to the parish authorities; in fifteenth-century Montpellier, people living in close proximity to suspected lepers delivered their accusations to the civic government.[130]

More than forty years later, on 3 September 1586, the parish of Saint-Maclou, Rouen, paid two physicians, Masters Guillaume Guerente and Pierre

---

122 *Regestrum*, 538; *Register*, 614. See pp. 70–2 above.

123 AN, Paris, S4889B, dossier 13, last document, fo. 1r.

124 Huneycutt, *Matilda of Scotland*, 105.

125 Demaitre, *Leprosy*, 155. See also pp. 130–1.

126 Ibid. 130.

127 'de morbo lepre suspectus': ADSM, G6606. In the Pas-de-Calais, leprosy examinations tended to take place in the *leprosaria* of sizeable towns: Bourgeois, *Lépreux*, 27.

128 ADSM, G6606.

129 Ibid.

130 Dumas, 'Bien public', forthcoming.

Columbel, and a surgeon, Master Claude Collumbel, 6 *livres* for examining Madeleine Morin, the wife of Jehan Prévost, and their daughter Robine Le Prévost, to ascertain whether the two women were leprous. The cases were confirmed, and it was established that the women needed to be separated from the healthy. Again, the parish oversaw the judgement, and here it took responsibility for maintaining those who had been diagnosed with leprosy. The parish paid the women 24 *livres* for their sustenance, and pledged to pay them a further 30 *sous* per week. It also arranged for the *leprosarium* of Saint-Léger-du-Bourg-Denis, to which the parish traditionally sent its lepers, to be rebuilt to accommodate them.[131] At the time the leper house was described as 'ruined and destroyed', suggesting that it had not served its function for several decades.[132] The parish accounts for the year 1589 reveal that Robine Le Prévost was still being supported three years later, receiving 14 *sous* 4 *deniers* per week for her food.[133] It would appear that her mother, Madeleine Morin, had died by that time; yet Robine was still receiving the same weekly sum from the parish in 1591.[134] The leprosy of a mother and her daughter in this case could reflect heredity, although, if they did both suffer from leprosy, the disease could well have been transmitted between them through close daily contact. From the fourteenth century, leprosy did come to be viewed as a hereditary disease by medical writers: Guy de Chauliac listed 'a stain in the generation' as one of the primary causes of leprosy.[135]

As in other parts of Europe, the process of diagnosis in Rouen varied and changed over time. While medical practitioners and parish authorities could play key roles in this procedure, by the sixteenth century lepers themselves were credited with the ability to identify the signs and symptoms of the disease. Physicians and surgeons evidently charged high fees for examining a suspected leper; an examination by leprosy sufferers may have proved the more affordable option. By this time, it appears to have been customary to examine those suspected of having leprosy, suggesting that it was considered important to make a correct diagnosis and, perhaps, to protect the healthy from contagion and infection.

Shifting responses to leprosy in Rouen between the twelfth and fifteenth centuries reflect changing ideas and practices in the realms of medical care, diagnosis and public health provision in this period. Prior to the Black Death, efforts were already being made to prevent lepers from mixing with the non-

---

[131] For the leper house of Saint-Léger-du-Bourg-Denis see pp. 79, 80 above.
[132] ruinée et desmollye': ADSM, G6897, fos 89r–92v; Charles de Robillard de Beaurepaire, *Inventaire-Sommaire des Archives Départementales antérieures à 1790: Seine-Inférieure, archives ecclésiastiques – Série G*, v (nos 6221–7370), Rouen 1892, 287–8; Fournée, 'Maladreries', 111.
[133] ADSM, G6898, fo. 53v.
[134] ADSM, G6902, fos 92v–93r.
[135] Demaitre, *Leprosy*, 158.

leprous, whether as a result of concerns about contagion, or because of a perception that the appropriate place for lepers was the *leprosarium*, where they could receive physical and spiritual care. The bodily care of the leprous was shaped by medical theory, particularly the concepts of the humours and the non-naturals, and reveals that concerted efforts were made to alleviate the suffering of the lepers and to make them comfortable. Records of diagnostic examinations highlight the importance of identifying cases of the disease, and shed light on the activities of medical practitioners in Rouen. Above all, the evidence from this city reveals that, although the Black Death was undoubtedly a turning point in the understanding of disease in medieval Europe, ideas about contagion and infection evolved over a much longer period. Responses to leprosy were diverse and fluctuating, and indicate that, as early as the thirteenth century, contemporaries reacted to the disease as an entity, as well as to its sufferers.

5

Leprosy and the Religious Culture of Rouen

Religious worship was a central aspect of life in the medieval leper house. Pious activities were intended to ensure the spiritual wellbeing of the leprous and non-leprous members of the resident community, as well as its benefactors. The extant architectural remains of the churches of Saint-Jacques and Saint-Thomas at Mont-aux-Malades, and the chapel of Saint-Julien at Salle-aux-Puelles, facilitate an understanding of the multiple spiritual functions of these institutions. Within these churches, masses were said, candles were lit on behalf of benefactors and many other observances took place. The churches also housed liturgical objects and relics, and they, and the cemeteries associated with them, were sites of burial. The popularity of Mont-aux-Malades as a site of lay piety was in large part due to the flourishing cult of St Thomas Becket from the late twelfth century. Yet the presence of lepers was also important: donations to Mont-aux-Malades and Salle-aux-Puelles were motivated by the perception that lepers' prayers were particularly efficacious, and the view that this group should be supported in pursuing a religious vocation. Liturgical practice and piety at these two institutions reflect their monastic organisation, as well as the understanding that the care of the body was inseparable from that of the soul.

Liturgical spaces at Mont-aux-Malades and Salle-aux-Puelles

Rouen's two major leper houses were equipped with fine churches, reflecting their high status as institutions, and the importance of liturgy within the daily routine of their communities. At Mont-aux-Malades, the first priory church, dedicated to St James, was built in the first part of the twelfth century, probably by about 1140, by which time Augustinian canons had probably been installed at the *leprosarium*.[1] The church was constructed near the Roman road between Rouen and Lillebonne (now rue Louis Pasteur). Although only four bays of the nave remain standing today, this was undoubtedly a large and impressive church: the extant part of the nave measures 18.5 by 6.5 metres (*see* Figure 5).[2] The nave was flanked by side-aisles; these, and the

---

[1] Georges Lanfry, 'L'Église Saint-Jacques du Mont-aux-Malades: bref résumé d'histoire', *Bulletin de la Commission des Antiquités de la Seine Maritime* xxvii (1968–9), 167; Lucien Musset, *Normandie romane*, II: *La Haute-Normandie*, Yonne 1974, 29.

[2] Musset, *Normandie romane*, 29.

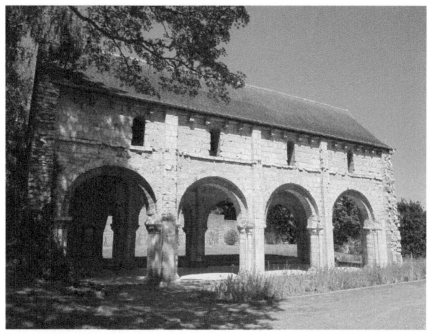

Figure 5. The priory church of Saint-Jacques at Mont-aux-Malades.

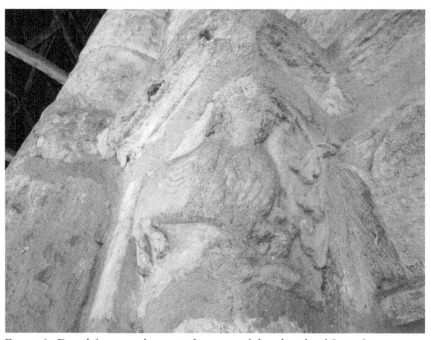

Figure 6. Detail from a column in the nave of the church of Saint-Jacques at Mont-aux-Malades.

semi-circular choir and the apse, have now disappeared. There was also a bell tower, meaning that the church's silhouette would have stood out prominently to those travelling along the road.[3]

The church's simple rounded arches, small windows and heavy stone columns decorated with carvings clearly reflect the Romanesque style, supporting its construction in the early twelfth century.[4] Lucien Musset argued that the church is one of the finest examples of Norman Romanesque masonry.[5] The church was damaged during the siege of Rouen by King Henry IV of France in 1591, when the side-aisles were destroyed and the nave converted into an arsenal.[6] A watercolour from the eighteenth century reveals that additional structures that no longer survive were attached to the church at that time.[7]

The extant fabric of the church of Saint-Jacques indicates that it was originally richly decorated. The capitals of the columns of the nave are ornamented with stone carvings, depicting foliage and animals (see Figure 6). Traces of a red-brown colour can be discerned on these capitals, which may suggest that the church's interior was originally brightly painted. Such decoration would not have been unusual: in England, paint traces are extant in the leper church of St Nicholas, Harbledown, outside Canterbury, and in that of the leper house near Wimborne, Dorset. Other English churches catering for lepers were furnished with decorative wall hangings.[8]

The chapel of Saint-Julien at Petit-Quevilly, which served the leprous women of Salle-aux-Puelles from the 1180s, with its wall-paintings depicting the Infancy of Christ (see Figure 4), certainly had a colourful interior.[9] Like the church of Saint-Jacques at Mont-aux-Malades, the chapel of Saint-Julien (see Figure 3), built in the early 1160s by Henry II as part of his manor at Quevilly, has a rich scheme of sculptural ornamentation (for details of the carving of the doorways, see Figure 7). The capitals of the columns supporting the arcade and the vaults bear carvings of fantastic animals, grotesque faces, foliage and geometric designs.[10]

The priory church of Saint-Thomas at Mont-aux-Malades, which replaced the church of Saint-Jacques, was constructed by Henry II to the north of

---

3   Ibid. 29–30; Deschamps, 'Léproseries', 34.

4   Lindy Grant, *Architecture and society in Normandy, 1120–1270*, New Haven 2005, 57.

5   Musset, *Normandie romane*, 30.

6   Lanfry, 'L'Église', 169.

7   Facsimile copy of an unsigned watercolour, by Adolphe Jean Duboc, showing the priory church of Saint-Jacques at Mont-aux-Malades and other buildings, undated (eighteenth century): Direction Régionale des Affaires Culturelles de Haute-Normandie/Service Régional de l'Inventaire Général, Rouen, dossier 76 INV 527 (Mont-Saint-Aignan).

8   Rawcliffe, *Leprosy*, 341.

9   Stratford, 'The wall-paintings', 51.

10   Étienne-Steiner, *Chapelle Saint-Julien*, 6.

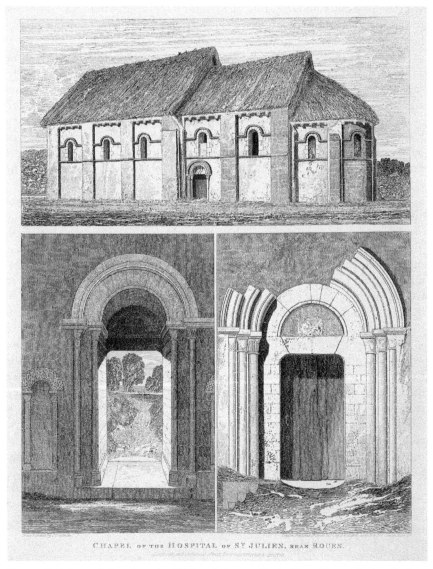

CHAPEL OF THE HOSPITAL OF ST JULIEN, NEAR ROUEN.

Figure 7. View of the chapel of Saint-Julien at Petit-Quevilly, with detailed views of doorways. Etching by John Sell Cotman, 1820.

Saint-Jacques in about 1174.[11] Since the transition to Gothic architecture began about 1140 with the construction of the abbey church of Saint-Denis near Paris, Saint-Thomas is a particularly late example of Romanesque architecture.[12] This church, which incorporates building phases from the seventeenth and nineteenth centuries, still serves as a parish church today.[13] The twelfth-century nave and choir are extant, and reveal that the church was built on a scale similar to that of Saint-Jacques. From the exterior a row of nine windows above the nave is visible. These are situated below a cornice decorated with a row of sculpted grotesques or animal heads, reminiscent of the stone carving at both the church of Saint-Jacques and the chapel of Saint-Julien (see Figure 8).[14] The side-aisles of the church of Saint-Thomas were added at a later date, presumably in the thirteenth century. The external walls of the side-aisles reflect the Gothic style, through the pointed arches of the windows, their trefoil ornamentation and the gargoyles flanking each window.[15] It appears, therefore, that the church of Saint-Thomas was enlarged in the thirteenth century, perhaps as a result of the church's increasing popularity as a focus of piety. The multiple donations received by Mont-aux-Malades from Rouen's burgesses at this time would have financed the building work.

Altars, lights and chantry chapels

As in many other churches, there were several different altars inside the church of Saint-Thomas at Mont-aux-Malades. Donation charters from the first half of the thirteenth century, on behalf of Nicholas Pigache, mayor of Rouen in 1208–9 and 1219–20 (issued in July 1219) and Matilda Le Changeur (issued in 1228), reveal the existence of two altars, dedicated to St Mary Magdalene and the Holy Trinity.[16] Presumably the church also housed an altar honouring St Thomas Becket. Referring to an inventory of Mont-aux-Malades' relics made in 1610, Pierre Langlois mentions the 'master altar' and the altar of St Vincent.[17] Between 1206 and 1218 the burgess Ralph the Jew made a gift 'to God and St Mary and St Thomas the Martyr' of Mont-aux-Malades, which could suggest that there was also an altar dedicated to

---

11 Lanfry, 'L'Église', 168.

12 Grant, Architecture, 58.

13 Deschamps, 'Léproseries', 41, 44; Lanfry, 'L'Église', 169.

14 Deschamps, 'Léproseries', 41; Étienne-Steiner, Chapelle Saint-Julien, 5.

15 Grant, Architecture, 57.

16 Appendix 2, nos 57 (Matilda Le Changeur), 62 (Nicholas Pigache).

17 'maître-autel': Langlois, Histoire, 365.

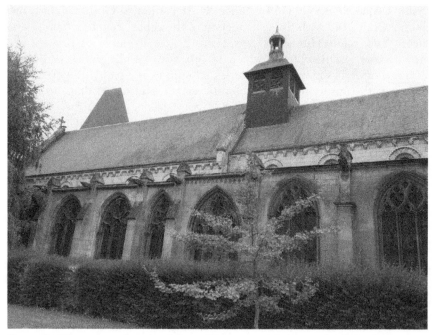

Figure 8. The priory church of Saint-Thomas at Mont-aux-Malades (side view).

the Virgin Mary inside this church, although his charter could alternatively allude to the altar of Mary Magdalene.[18]

The fact that monastic churches like that of Mont-aux-Malades offered a variety of altars dedicated to different saints, each of which required lighting, may have particularly encouraged the endowment of candles.[19] Provision for the burning of candles at altars was especially pronounced among liturgical practices at Mont-aux-Malades, and underlines the links between the leper house community and Rouen's lay population. Four charters marking such arrangements were issued in the late twelfth and the first part of the thirteenth century; three of these date from a period of less than a decade (1219–28). This suggests that provision for candles was a particularly strong trend in lay piety in the first third of the thirteenth century. Indeed, David Postles argues that the decrees of the Fourth Lateran Council (1215) 'were a stimulus to internal piety which was expressed through voluntary lay benefactions for lights'.[20]

[18] 'deo et beate marie et Sancto Thome martyri de monte Leprosorum': appendix 2, no. 78.

[19] Postles, 'Lamps', 97, 105, 106–7.

[20] Ibid. 113.

The lighting of leper house chapels particularly served to illuminate the eucharist, making it possible for the leprous to see the body and blood of Christ.[21] Candles were also essential to ensuring that the church was a place where people could be emotionally and spiritually uplifted by light.[22] The endowment of lights in leper house churches, therefore, facilitated the spiritual care of lepers.[23] Candles were also associated with healing: at shrines it was common for a sick person to offer a candle containing a folded wick the length of their body.[24]

In the last quarter of the twelfth century, for the salvation of his soul, Matthew de Neuville donated a measure of salt and 6 *sous* of rent to Mont-aux-Malades, 'towards the lighting of the church of St Thomas the Martyr'.[25] While this gift did not stipulate that a particular altar should be lit or a specific feast day be observed, later gifts concerning candles were more specific. In July 1219 Nicholas Pigache donated a rent of 40 *sous* of Tours to fund a lamp burning constantly before the altar of St Mary Magdalene in the church of Saint-Thomas.[26] In July 1226 Peter and Avicia de Saint-Jacques gave 5 *sous* annual rent to Mont-aux-Malades, with the agreement of Prior William (1222–33) to retain ½ *livre* of the rent to fund a candle burning once a year in perpetuity, on the feast (29 July) of St Martha the Martyr, sister of St Mary Magdalene.[27] Although this was presented as a gift in perpetual alms, 5 *sous* was a very small, nominal sum, and Mont-aux-Malades itself gave the couple 40 *sous* of Tours in return.[28] It appears that the endowment of candles was inexpensive; nonetheless, the gifts discussed here were made by high-status burgesses.[29] In 1228 Matilda Le Changeur, a member of another leading Rouen family, donated 22 *sous* annual rent in perpetuity, to illuminate the altar of the Holy Trinity in the church of Saint-Thomas. Like Matthew de Neuville, she made the gift for her salvation alone, not mentioning the souls of family members, which implies that there was a particularly strong link between candles and personal salvation.[30]

The association of St Mary Magdalene and St Martha with the endowments of candles reflects the popularity of these female saints at this time. At least sixty-nine leper houses established in England by about 1300 were dedicated to Mary Magdalene, just less than one third of those whose dedi-

---

[21] Rawcliffe, *Leprosy*, 341.

[22] See ibid.

[23] See ibid. n. 183 on 'the therapeutic value of *seeing* the Eucharist'.

[24] Postles, 'Lamps', 103.

[25] 'ad lumen ecclesie sancti thome martiris': appendix 2, no. 59.

[26] Ibid. no. 62.

[27] Ibid. no. 70.

[28] Ibid.

[29] See Postles, 'Lamps', 97, 105, 113, and Rawcliffe, *Leprosy*, 341–2.

[30] Appendix 2, no. 57.

cation is known.[31] Mary was closely associated with repentance and healing, through her penitence for her sins as a prostitute and her use of ointment to prepare Christ's body for burial.[32] Although it was not expected that lepers would be healed at *leprosaria*, the example set by Mary Magdalene in terms of tending the bodies of the sick was highly appropriate for these institutions. She was also linked more specifically to leprosy: her Old Testament precursor was Miriam, sister of Moses, who was struck with leprosy for her sins.[33]

Martha was the sister of the two siblings Mary and Lazarus of Bethany, who gave Christ hospitality at Bethany.[34] St Ambrose identified her with the woman whose ceaseless menstrual flow was miraculously healed by Christ. Martha's ailment had signalled her impurity and had made her an outcast, indicating why she herself was associated with the plight of lepers.[35] During the Middle Ages a legend developed which equated Mary of Bethany with Mary Magdalene, and proposed that Mary, Martha and Lazarus together evangelised the region of Provence.[36] The English *leprosarium* at Sherburn, founded in about 1181 by Hugh le Puiset, bishop of Durham (1153–95), which was comparable to Mont-aux-Malades in size and status, was jointly dedicated to Mary, Martha and Lazarus, evidencing the association of Martha, alongside Mary Magdalene and Lazarus, with leprosy.[37]

It appears that a separate chantry chapel was established around the altar of St Mary Magdalene in the church of Saint-Thomas in the thirteenth century. Nicholas Pigache's endowment in July 1219 included a gift of 10 *livres* of Tours to support a priest to celebrate mass daily, at the altar of St Mary Magdalene in the presence of female lepers, for the salvation of Nicholas, his wife, parents and other ancestors.[38] This arrangement would have been intended to benefit the souls of the leprous women at Mont-aux-Malades, as well as those of Nicholas Pigache and his family. Archbishop Eudes Rigaud's visitation records, at 1 April 1264, refer to the secular priest celebrating mass 'in the Pigache chapel', indicating that by this point the Pigache family had established a separate chapel around this altar, served by a private priest.[39] Chantries were a distinctive feature of lay piety from the thirteenth century, reflecting the belief that private intercession helped to

[31] Rawcliffe, *Leprosy*, 120.

[32] Ibid. 119–21.

[33] Ibid. 119.

[34] David H. Farmer, *The Oxford dictionary of saints*, 5th edn, Oxford 2003, 349.

[35] Rawcliffe, *Leprosy*, 119.

[36] Farmer, *Oxford dictionary*, 350, 357–8.

[37] Rawcliffe, *Leprosy*, 119.

[38] Appendix 2, no. 62.

[39] 'in capella Pyage': *Regestrum*, 513; *Register*, 585.

reduce the pain of purgatory.[40] A chantry consisted of the establishment of a mass to be performed at a specific altar, and did not necessarily entail the construction of a chapel. However, chapels were built by wealthy benefactors to accommodate their chantries, with a view to the celebration of masses on their behalf in perpetuity.[41] The first chantry chapels in France were located in cathedrals (including Amiens cathedral, Rouen cathedral and Notre-Dame, Paris), but they did not begin to be widespread in Europe until the second half of the thirteenth century.[42] By the early fourteenth century, chantries were being established in Rouen's parish churches: in 1304 John Hardi provided in his testament for a chapel and priest to be established in his parish church, Saint-Martin-du-Pont, for his salvation and that of his friends and successors.[43] The chapel founded by the Pigache family at Mont-aux-Malades was an early example of a chantry chapel, particularly in light of its location inside a leper house church.

Liturgical objects and relics

Although little information survives concerning the furnishings of the churches of Saint-Thomas and Saint-Julien and the objects that they held, it can be assumed that both churches housed liturgical books (including obituaries), gold and silver ornaments, fine vestments and wall-hangings, altarpieces, relics and reliquaries. Such objects played a role in the mass and other divine services, and were a focus of piety and veneration. They also demonstrated the material wealth of the community. While Archbishop Rigaud complained of the absence of liturgical books at certain religious houses, such as the priory of Gasny (a dependency of the abbey of Saint-Ouen, Rouen) and the Augustinian chapter of Saint-Mellon de Pontoise, he made no such complaints when visiting Mont-aux-Malades or Salle-aux-Puelles.[44] This suggests that, in the mid-thirteenth century at least, both communities did possess such essential books as the Bible, psalters and antiphonaries.[45]

In 1240 Peter de Collemezzo ordered the dean of Rouen to make an inventory of the books, revenues, vestments and other ornaments in the

---

[40] Howard Colvin, 'The origin of chantries', *Journal of Medieval History* xxvi (2000), 163, 168–9; David Crouch, 'The origin of chantries: some further Anglo-Norman evidence', *Journal of Medieval History* xxvii (2001), 159–60.

[41] Simon Roffey, *Chantry chapels and medieval strategies for the afterlife*, Stroud 2008, 16–17.

[42] Colvin, 'Origin', 164–5; Doquang, 'Status and the soul', 99–100; Roffey, *Chantry chapels*, 18.

[43] Appendix 2, no. 43.

[44] *Regestrum*, 240, 391, 494–5; *Register*, 266, 446, 563; Davis, *Holy bureaucrat*, 89.

[45] Cf. Davis, *Holy bureaucrat*, 89.

church of Moulineaux, a dependency of Salle-aux-Puelles.[46] The archbishop's expectation that a small parish church would hold a number of such objects strongly suggests that the wealthy monastic churches of Mont-aux-Malades and Salle-aux-Puelles had many such possessions. Such an assumption is further supported by the rich material holdings of the parish churches of late medieval Norwich, a city of comparable size and prosperity to Rouen.[47] Furthermore, a number of modest leprosaria in England had sizeable collections of liturgical items, such as St Mary Magdalen, Sprowston, which possessed silver-gilt chalices, processionals, vestments and other objects in the mid-fourteenth century, and the house at Gaywood, outside King's Lynn, from which several items were stolen in the 1450s.[48]

Relics, providing a direct and tangible link with the saints, were particularly treasured possessions. Much as benefactors amassed prayers on behalf of their souls from a range of religious communities, the accumulation of relics by churches resulted in a treasury of spiritually potent objects, which were sometimes believed to bring about healing.[49] Relics straddled the boundary between human being and object. They were the vestiges of humans, as the body parts or former possessions of saints, and were understood to be able to act with intention.[50] In March 1267/8 Rouen's La Madeleine hospital received relics of St Mary Magdalene from Louis IX, delivered by the king's friend, Archbishop Rigaud.[51] In his history of Mont-aux-Malades, Pierre Langlois refers to an inventory of 1610 listing the relics held in the church of Saint-Thomas at that date, but no longer present by the mid-nineteenth century.[52] Housed in many precious reliquaries of silver, silver-gilt and gilded wood, these included the whole left arm of St Vincent, relics of St Denis and his companion martyrs, and relics of many other saints, including Hugh, archbishop of Rouen (c. 732–40). Most important, one reliquary contained a bone of St Thomas Becket and fragments of his stole, goblet, rochet and hair-shirt. There were also fourteen frames containing relics of various saints and relics brought back from the Holy Land.[53]

Although it is impossible to know exactly when these relics and reliquaries were acquired prior to 1610, Langlois's account conveys the wealth that they represented, both materially and spiritually, and the manner in which the church of Saint-Thomas was populated with precious objects. As well as

---

[46] Appendix 2, no. 67(a).

[47] See Hill, *Women and religion*, especially plates.

[48] Rawcliffe, *Leprosy*, 340–1.

[49] On the potency of relics see, for example, Patrick J. Geary, *Furta sacra: thefts of relics in the central Middle Ages*, revised edn, Princeton, NJ 1990, 32–4.

[50] On the agency of relics as objects see Roberta Gilchrist, *Medieval life: archaeology and the life course*, Woodbridge 2012, 217–18.

[51] *Regestrum*, 597; *Register*, 687.

[52] Langlois, *Histoire*, 361–6. I have not located the 1610 inventory.

[53] Ibid.

enhancing the environment in which the lepers, canons and lay brethren worshipped, the relics, particularly those of Thomas Becket, attracted people from outside the community to the church and encouraged donations. In England, where most *leprosaria* were modest foundations, large relic collections were rare, although in 1391 the residents of St Bartholomew, Oxford, claimed that Oriel College had removed several of their relics, including a piece of the skin of St Bartholomew.[54] Relics and reliquaries were more likely to be associated with large, high-status *leprosaria* like Mont-aux-Malades, and added a further dimension to liturgical practice and piety.

Burial and commemoration

Leper houses were sites of burial and the commemoration of souls, for not only their residents but also their benefactors. From the thirteenth century, as the doctrine of purgatory became increasingly well-established, arrangements for commemorative prayers and masses multiplied, since it was believed that these rites would reduce the length of time that the soul lingered in purgatory. A visible tombstone within a church would evoke the memory of the deceased person, and remind the living to pray for them.[55] Much light has been shed on burial practices at monasteries, hospitals and *leprosaria* by archaeologists studying the cemeteries associated with these institutions.[56] Although there have been no recent archaeological studies of Rouen's *leprosaria*, an extensive excavation of the *leprosarium* of Saint-Thomas at Aizier (Eure), a village mid-way between Rouen and Le Havre, was completed between 1998 and 2010.[57] Aizier's leper house was founded before 1227, probably about 1173–80, on land belonging to the abbey of Fécamp.[58] A number of burials have been excavated around the chapel, particularly in the area immediately north of it.[59]

---

[54] Carole Rawcliffe has suggested that the size of St Bartholomew's relic collection may have been exaggerated in the context of the dispute with Oriel College: *Leprosy*, 340 n. 177.

[55] See Roffey, *Chantry chapels*, 16, 19–20.

[56] For *leprosaria* see, for example, Magilton, Lee and Boylston, *'Lepers outside the gate'*; Cécile Paresys, 'Saint-Ladre de Reims, un cimetière de lépreux?', in Tabuteau, *Étude des lépreux*, 111–22; and Damien Jeanne, 'Quelles Problématiques pour la mort du lépreux? Sondages archéologiques du cimetière de Saint-Nicolas-de-la-Chesnaie – Bayeux', *AN* xlvii (1997), 69–90.

[57] See http://www.unicaen.fr/crahm/spip.php?article120&lang=fr (accessed 21 July 2012), and Niel and Truc, 'La Chapelle Saint-Thomas d'Aizier', 47–107.

[58] Niel and Truc, 'La Chapelle Saint-Thomas d'Aizier', 50–1; Luc Bonnin, 'Saint-Thomas d'Aizier: un exemple de projet de valorisation d'un site archéologique de léproserie médiévale', in Tabuteau, *Étude des lépreux*, 35–6.

[59] Niel and Truc, 'La Chapelle Saint-Thomas d'Aizier', 74–5.

Documentary evidence suggests that several high-status benefactors were buried at Mont-aux-Malades in the twelfth, thirteenth and fourteenth centuries, reflecting practices at many other monastic houses, hospitals and leper houses in France and England. Such burials consolidated relationships between aristocratic families and monastic houses. The space assigned to burials was significant, with interment within the chapter house or near the high altar particularly valued.[60] The cartulary of Chichester cathedral reveals that Richard, son of the clerk, his mother and her husband were buried in the cemetery of the *leprosarium* of St James's, Chichester, by the end of the twelfth century or beginning of the thirteenth century. Excavations at St James's have uncovered a walled area in the cemetery containing two adult non-leprous female skeletons, who evidently received a privileged burial, in what was possibly a mortuary house or even a chantry chapel within the *leprosarium*'s church. John Magilton suggests that these women, one of whom was apparently wearing a headdress (evidenced by pins around the skull), were benefactors 'or otherwise locally renowned for their piety'.[61]

While monasteries received substantial endowments from the founders and patrons whom they buried, from the late twelfth century, lay individuals from more modest backgrounds, who were not significant benefactors, increasingly arranged their burial at monastic houses through *cum corpore* grants. This new trend, which peaked in the early thirteenth century, coincided with the emergence of the newer orders, especially the Augustinians, whose foundations provided new, more affordable opportunities for burial.[62] At first glance, the benefit to a monastic community of burying a deceased lay person's body is unclear. However, these burials provided an opportunity for the monastic house to demonstrate its usefulness and importance in the locality, and strengthened its links with lay society. Although the burial of high-status lay individuals undoubtedly achieved these goals, that of lower status lay people was also of considerable value towards these ends. In turn, lay people who found a place of burial at a monastery benefited from the intercessory prayers of the religious and, in some cases, a prestigious place of burial.[63]

One would expect that the canons of Mont-aux-Malades would be buried in the church of Saint-Thomas. Indeed, the tombstone of Peter Restout, canon of Saint-Thomas and rector of the church of Saint-Jacques, who died

[60] Danielle Westerhof, *Death and the noble body in medieval England*, Woodbridge 2008, 66–8.

[61] John Magilton, 'The cemetery', in Magilton, Lee and Boylston, *'Lepers outside the gate'*, 84–6, 127–8. Although other burials of women with pins around their heads have been excavated at English nunneries, Magilton argues that the Chichester woman was not necessarily a professed religious.

[62] David Postles, 'Monastic burials of non-patronal lay benefactors', *Journal of Ecclesiastical History* xlvii (1996), 625, 630–1.

[63] Ibid. 624–5, 631–2.

in 1380, was located in the principal aisle of Saint-Thomas in the mid-nine-teenth century.[64] The earliest benefactor of Mont-aux-Malades who arranged to be buried there was Roscelin, son of Clarembaud, Henry II's chamberlain and a royal justice.[65] Between 1154 and 1164 Roscelin founded the parish church of Saint-Gilles at Mont-aux-Malades, endowed it with 7 *livres* of rent, and arranged for one of the leper house's canons to serve in it. He estab-lished that 'because I am its [the church's] founder, I have given up my body to be buried there'.[66] The wording of Roscelin's act suggests that he expected to be buried inside the church, like high-status benefactors elsewhere, who were often buried before the altar.[67] It was appropriate for him to be buried in the church because it was a testament to his piety and generosity in founding it. Furthermore, he could expect that the canon of Mont-aux-Malades who served in the church would regularly intercede for his soul.

In the thirteenth and early fourteenth century, other distinguished patrons were buried at Mont-aux-Malades. Nicholas de la Commune, a cleric, arranged for his burial in his testament, witnessed in a *vidimus* of the official of Rouen in 1262.[68] Few testaments from this period are recorded, suggesting that there could have been many similar arrangements for burial about which no evidence now survives.[69] Nicholas also donated a silver cup, which could have been a liturgical object that was subsequently used or displayed in the church of Saint-Thomas. Similar objects were bequeathed to family members in later medieval Douai (northern France), suggesting that Nicholas's gift, as well as his arrangements for burial, indicate a close personal relationship with the community at Mont-aux-Malades.[70] Indeed, the prior of the leper house was an executor of the testament, and the prior's seal was attached to the *vidimus* of the document.

A high-status couple, Laurence Chamberlain and his wife Matilda, were also buried at Mont-aux-Malades. The carved tombstone of Matilda (*see* Figure 2), who died in 1293, is extant in the church of Saint-Thomas today. It is now embedded within one of the walls, but its exact original loca-tion is unknown.[71] The tombstone of Laurence (d. 1304) was also appar-ently housed in the church; however, by the mid-nineteenth century it had disappeared.[72] Laurence was Louis IX's *panetier royal*, an official of the royal

---

[64] Langlois, *Histoire*, 358.

[65] For Roscelin's status as a royal justice see appendix 2, no. 24 (act of Geoffrey II, dean of Rouen).

[66] 'quia fundator illius sum, meum corpus ibi sepeliri deuoui': ibid. no. 95.

[67] See Postles, 'Monastic burials', 634.

[68] Appendix 2, no. 60.

[69] See Rawcliffe, *Leprosy*, 262.

[70] Martha C. Howell, 'Fixing movables: gifts by testament in late medieval Douai', *Past & Present* cl (1996), 6, 8.

[71] Langlois, *Histoire*, 97, 356; Deschamps, 'Léproseries', 42, and 'L'Abbé Cochet', i. 31.

[72] Langlois, *Histoire*, 358.

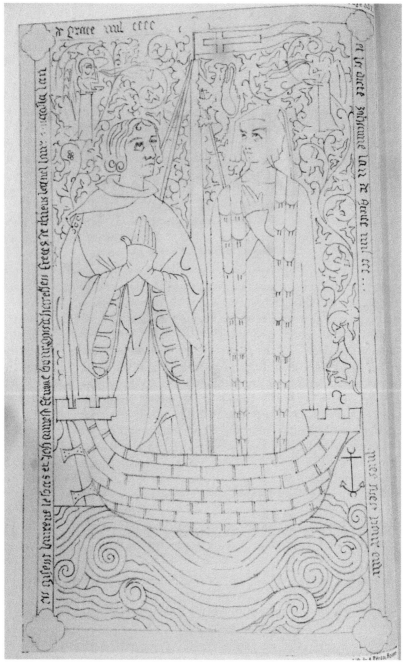

Figure 9. Tombstone of Laurence Lebas (d. 1400) and his wife Jeanne
(d. 1389), located in the chapel of the Holy Virgin in the church of Saint-
Thomas at Mont-aux-Malades in the mid-nineteenth century. Lithograph
by A. Péron, in Langlois, *Histoire*, frontispiece.

household in charge of bakers and bakeries, at Rouen, and became lord of Saint-Aignan, the area in the immediate vicinity of Mont-aux-Malades, in 1259.[73] He was a very generous patron, granting the *leprosarium* the fief of Saint-Aignan in 1289, with Matilda's consent.[74] The couple's decision to be buried at Mont-aux-Malades may reflect their attachment to the local area, as well as a belief that burial in proximity to other patrons and members of the leper house community would be spiritually beneficial. They no doubt also sought the lepers' intercessory prayers for their souls, prayers that would have been encouraged by the visible presence of their tombs within the church.[75] Nonetheless, it is unlikely that they were buried near deceased lepers. While patrons had the privilege of being buried within the church of Saint-Thomas, the leprous were probably interred in the cemetery outside the church.[76]

At the turn of the fifteenth century, another couple, Laurence Lebas (d. 1400) and his wife Jeanne (d. 1389), burgesses of the sea port of Harfleur (dép. Seine-Maritime, canton Gonfreville-l'Orcher), were buried in the church of Saint-Thomas. In the mid-nineteenth century, their shared tombstone was located in the chapel of the Holy Virgin beneath a trap door in the floor.[77] The tomb slab (*see* Figure 9) described them as 'freres de chiens [céans]' ('brothers of this house'), which may suggest that the couple entered the leper house as lay brethren.[78] It depicted two figures standing upright in a small boat on the sea, linking Laurence and Jeanne to their coastal home town and also, perhaps, symbolising the Christian journey to heaven after death, or the moment of the resurrection.[79]

Although anniversary masses were fundamental to the commemorative expectations of lay patrons, direct evidence for their performance at Mont-aux-Malades and Salle-aux-Puelles is scant. Commemorative activities at the two leper houses would certainly have remembered deceased leprous residents. In England, many of the more affluent *leprosaria* made such arrangements, which were often very elaborate. At Colchester's leper house, for example, the master visited the deceased leper's grave after each mass, and every leper had to say 100 *Pater Nosters* for the deceased daily for one month.[80]

---

[73] Ibid. 97.

[74] Appendix 2, no. 52(b). Laurence and Matilda's patronage for Mont-aux-Malades is discussed at pp. 45–7 above.

[75] See Postles, 'Monastic burials', 625.

[76] See Rawcliffe, *Leprosy*, 262.

[77] Langlois, *Histoire*, 329, 357–8.

[78] Ibid. frontispiece, 357.

[79] See Langlois, *Histoire*, 357–8, and Gilchrist, *Medieval life*, 199.

[80] Rawcliffe, *Leprosy*, 342–3.

In terms of the commemoration of benefactors, at Mont-aux-Malades this is evidenced indirectly (and sometimes directly) by the numerous extant charters, and smaller number of testaments, favouring the *leprosarium*. Since most donors specified that they made their gifts for the salvation of their souls and those of family members, they must have assumed that prayers would be performed in the leper house church on their behalf, either on their anniversary or at another appropriate time, such as the Feast of the Dead on 2 November.[81] In a charter of 1174–1200 for Mont-aux-Malades, Ralph and William d'Esneval specifically provided for an annual rent of 20 *sous* to be paid on their mother's anniversary.[82] This arrangement implies the brothers' belief that the delivery of the sum on this specific day would help to ensure her salvation. It also indicates their wish to honour her memory on this date.

The only two explicit requests for anniversary masses to be performed in the church itself at Mont-aux-Malades are contained in charters of Philip III and Philip IV, issued in August 1281 and December 1296 respectively. When donating the church of Saint-Martin at Fréville to Mont-aux-Malades, Philip III arranged for a canon of the leper house to celebrate mass daily on his behalf in Fréville's church: a mass of the Holy Spirit while he lived, and a mass of the dead after his death. He also arranged for his anniversary to be commemorated annually in the church of Mont-aux-Malades.[83] Fifteen years later Philip IV made very similar arrangements at the time of his gift of the church of Saint-Aignan: he required a daily mass on behalf of himself and his wife Jeanne in this church, and for the religious of Mont-aux-Malades to celebrate his and Jeanne's anniversaries in the *leprosarium*'s church following their deaths.[84] These royal provisions suggest that it was important to arrange frequent intercession at the exact site of a donation (here, the two dependent churches donated by these kings), and to reinforce this intercession through an anniversary mass. It is very likely that the anniversaries of other major benefactors were similarly honoured in the church at Mont-aux-Malades.

Such anniversaries would have been recorded in an obituary (memorial book), a volume held by a religious community and organised according to the liturgical calendar, listing under each day the names of individuals associated with the community who had died on that day, and often providing

---

[81] 'the expectation of the return in gift-exchange for salvific purposes was often unspecified, if generally understood: prayers for the benefactor and her or his kinship': Postles, 'Lamps', 112.

[82] Appendix 2, no. 77; Langlois, *Histoire*, 101.

[83] Appendix 2, no. 74(b).

[84] Ibid. no. 75(b).

details of their donations or other pious acts.[85] Such documents are rich in information about piety, commemoration, economic history and material culture.[86] Langlois refers to Mont-aux-Malades' 'old obituary', lost by the mid-nineteenth century.[87] The community at Salle-aux-Puelles also probably maintained an obituary. The fifteenth-century obituary of Rouen's La Madeleine hospital is extant, with its first entries written down between 1460 and 1467, and many later additions up to the eighteenth century.[88] It appears to contain many entries from an earlier memorial book, now lost, since it includes the names of individuals who can be definitively dated to the late twelfth and thirteenth centuries.[89] The medieval obituaries of a handful of *leprosaria* and hospitals in France and England are also extant, including those of the high-status 'Red Church' *leprosarium* outside Strasbourg, Le Popelin at Sens, Le Grand Beaulieu at Chartres, the Quinze-Vingts hospital for the blind in Paris, and the *leprosarium* of St Mary Magdalen, Gaywood (outside King's Lynn).[90] Many similar documents were presumably lost during the Reformation in England, the Revolution in France and other post-medieval periods of upheaval. The survival of obituaries associated with distinguished, wealthy leper communities like those of Chartres and Sens reinforces the likelihood that such documents were also a key feature of liturgical practice at Mont-aux-Malades and Salle-aux-Puelles.

There is little evidence for testaments favouring Rouen's *leprosaria* between the twelfth and fifteenth centuries. Indeed, the practice of drawing up testaments only became popular from the fourteenth century. A study of poverty in medieval Paris identified only thirty-two testaments issued by Parisian burgesses between 1200 and 1348, although there was also evidence for many other testaments no longer extant today.[91] For Douai, the number of extant testaments increases markedly in the later Middle Ages: before 1270 only

---

[85] See Charlotte A. Stanford, *Commemorating the dead in late medieval Strasbourg: the cathedral's 'Book of Donors' and its use (1320–1521)*, Farnham 2011, p. xv. Strasbourg's *Book of donors* is an unusually large obituary listing 7,803 identifiable persons.

[86] Ibid. esp. pp. xv, 1 and ch. i.

[87] Langlois, *Histoire*, 276.

[88] BM, Rouen, MS Y42. See Jean-Loup Lemaître, *Répertoire des documents nécrologiques français*, Paris 1980–7, i. 263, and Dubois, 'Les Rouennais'. Excerpts from the manuscript are printed in *Recueil des historiens*, xxiii. 415–16.

[89] Dubois, 'Les Rouennais', 9–11.

[90] Jean-Loup Lemaître, *Répertoire des documents nécrologiques français: troisième supplement (1993–2008)*, Paris 2008, 20–1 (Quinze-Vingts); *L'Obituaire de l'Hôpital des Quinze-Vingts de Paris*, ed. Jean-Loup Lemaître, Paris 2011; Carole Rawcliffe, 'Communities of the living and of the dead: hospital confraternities in the later Middle Ages', in Christopher Bonfield, Jonathan Reinarz and Teresa Huguet-Termes (eds), *Hospitals and communities, 1100–1960*, Oxford 2013, 125–54 (Gaywood *leprosarium*).

[91] Sharon Farmer, *Surviving poverty in medieval Paris: gender, ideology and the daily lives of the poor*, Ithaca, NY 2002, 171–2.

seventeen such documents are extant; forty testaments survive from 1303 to 1329; and a total of up to 4,000 testaments issued before 1500 are conserved in Douai's municipal archive. These documents became increasingly elaborate, with late medieval testators enumerating each of their worldly possessions and its intended destination, usually a friend or relative.[92]

There is archival evidence for five testaments relating to Mont-aux-Malades issued between the late twelfth and early fourteenth centuries. At the end of the twelfth century (in 1195 or 1198–1200), Giles, son of Stephen, son of Tehard, donated 60 *sous* of rent to Mont-aux-Malades in perpetual alms, for the salvation of his soul and those of his parents and ancestors, 'and especially for the soul of my brother Nicholas, as he set out in his testament and I agreed with him'.[93] Although the rent was due from Giles's own possessions (his house in the parish of Saint-Vincent, Rouen, and his fief in the district of Estopée), it appears likely that a portion of the sum had been provided originally by his brother Nicholas.[94] In 1252 William Le Sochon and his siblings Ansquetillus, Sanson and Lucia ratified the gift to Mont-aux-Malades made in the testament of their brother, William de Milloel, formerly clerk of Stephen de la Porte, *bailli* of Rouen (1247–54). William had donated his tenement in the parish of Saint-Laurent, Rouen, for the salvation of his soul.[95] This was a substantial donation; the clerk could have been inspired by the generosity of his master, Stephen de la Porte, who was a patron of the abbey of Le Bec.[96] The four siblings received 100 *sous* of Tours from Mont-aux-Malades in return for consenting to their brother's gift. In 1262 the official of Rouen issued a *vidimus* witnessing the testament of Nicholas de la Commune, the contents of which are discussed above. Nicholas de la Commune's original testament may have named additional beneficiaries: religious houses often had only the relevant parts of testaments copied for their records.[97] However, Nicholas's wish to be buried at Mont-aux-Malades suggests that he did prioritise the *leprosarium*.

The most detailed testaments date from the early years of the fourteenth century. That of John Hardi, of the parish of Saint-Martin-du-Pont, Rouen, issued in 1304, favours several *leprosaria* and hospitals in Rouen and its environs, including Mont-aux-Malades, Salle-aux-Puelles and La Madeleine hospital.[98] On 16 August 1302 Geoffrey Le Cras, of the parish of Pîtres (Eure,

---

[92] Howell, 'Fixing movables', 3–5, 6–7, 8.

[93] 'et maxime pro anima Nicholai fratris mei sicut ipse diuisit in testamento suo et ego ei pepigi': appendix 2, no. 28.

[94] Ibid.

[95] Ibid. no. 114.

[96] Joseph R. Strayer, *The administration of Normandy under Saint Louis*, Cambridge, MA 1932, repr. New York 1971, 97.

[97] Farmer, *Surviving*, 171.

[98] Appendix 2, no. 43.

canton Pont-de-l'Arche), drew up an extensive testament, including amongst its beneficiaries La Madeleine, Mont-aux-Malades and three *leprosaria* in the vicinity of Pîtres (at Pont-de-l'Arche, Pont-Saint-Pierre and Chant-d'Oisel).[99] It is likely that both men expected all the religious communities favoured in their testaments to pray for their souls and commemorate their anniversaries, thus amassing intercessory activity that would benefit their souls in purgatory.

The care of souls

The commemoration of souls was one of a number of activities in Rouen's *leprosaria* that focused upon the care of the souls of the living and the dead. François-Olivier Touati has examined the special religious status of lepers in the twelfth and thirteenth centuries, and the manner in which the *leprosarium* provided a setting for their conversion to and pursuit of a religious vocation.[100] Confession, preaching and the celebration of mass were intended both to ensure the health of the lepers' souls, and to reassure and comfort them: indeed, confession and preaching can be equated with the modern-day practice of counselling. There were many dimensions to the spiritual care of both the leprous and the non-leprous within the walls of Rouen's *leprosaria*: from the religious status of the residents, to the emphasis on enclosure and confinement, which were understood ultimately to liberate souls.

Proper spiritual facilities at *leprosaria* were provided for in the canons of the Third Lateran Council of 1179. The council's twenty-third canon instructed that groups of lepers were to have their own churches, cemeteries and priests. Although the decree stated that 'lepers cannot dwell with the healthy or come to church with others', it still clearly envisaged them as members of Christian society.[101] It ensured that lepers would have the essential facilities that they needed as Christians: a place of worship, a priest and a proper place of burial. Archbishop Rigaud carefully observed these requirements when he made arrangements to found a *leprosarium* at Aliermont (département Seine-Maritime, canton Envermeu), north of Rouen, early in his archbishopric. A bull of Pope Innocent IV (1243–54) from October 1248 reveals that Rigaud intended to grant a piece of land to the lepers of Aliermont for a house to be built there for them. He also planned to found a church there in his *villa*, and wished it to have land for a cemetery and a small lodging for its priest.[102] Aliermont was the site of one of the archbishop's eleven manor houses, and

---

[99] Ibid. no. 26.

[100] Touati, 'Les Léproseries aux XIIème et XIIIème siècles', 1–32.

[101] 'leprosis qui cum sanis habitare non possunt et ad ecclesiam cum aliis convenire': *Decrees of the ecumenical councils*, i. 222; Avril, 'Le IIIe Concile', 21–76.

[102] Appendix 2, no. 19(a).

Eudes visited the village many times.[103] Although the bull does not explicitly associate the *leprosarium* with the church, cemetery and priest's lodging, there is every indication that the archbishop was adhering to the tenets of the Third Lateran Council's decree in arranging for his new foundation.

Concern for the spiritual wellbeing of lepers was exhibited in Eudes Rigaud's statutes for Salle-aux-Puelles, drawn up in August 1249. This text states: 'Let them make their confessions often, and let them take communion at least four times in the year, that is, on the birth of the Lord, on the fifth feast before Easter [Maundy Thursday], at Easter and at Pentecost.'[104] Although these instructions testify to the importance of spiritual observances at Salle-aux-Puelles, it is worth noting that they occupy only a small section of the statutes, which deal with many other issues such as diet, dress, bloodletting and living communally.[105] These more practical matters were considered as important as spiritual affairs to ensuring the proper functioning of Salle-aux-Puelles as a religious community, essential to the leprous women's pursuit of their vocation. The record of the subsequent visit to Salle-aux-Puelles by the archbishop, on 9 December 1258, states that 'They always sing Matins in the middle of the night, for which the sisters rise when they wish to, but they cannot be forced to do this.'[106] The performance of this midnight liturgy demonstrates that the daily timetable at Salle-aux-Puelles was highly structured around religious observances. Nonetheless, participation in this particular liturgy, which involved interrupting the night's sleep, was voluntary as far as the leprous sisters were concerned. This suggests that the women's physical condition was taken into account in terms of their liturgical obligations, much as the sick lying in monastic infirmaries were excused from participation in the daily routine of services.

Rouen's *leprosaria* were in many respects sites of confinement and enclosure, a characteristic closely linked to the care of souls. Imprisonment was a key concept in medieval Christianity, in particular shaping practices of monasticism and asceticism. Incarceration was associated with both purgation (atoning for one's sins) and the attainment of spiritual liberation and redemption through suffering in confinement.[107] Enclosure and confinement also played an important practical role in monastic houses, where it was considered essential to prevent apostasy and the infiltration of lay people into the cloister, and to discipline religious who disobeyed the monastic

103 Davis, *Holy bureaucrat*, 46–8.

104 'Confessiones suas frequenter faciant, et communicent ad minus quater in anno, videlicet in natali Domini, quinta feria ante pascha, in pascha, et in penthecoste': *Regestrum*, 102; *Register*, 117.

105 *Regestrum*, 101–2; *Regestrum*, 116–17.

106 'Semper dicuntur matutine media nocte, ad quas surgunt sorores quando volunt, nec possunt ad hoc compelli': *Regestrum*, 325; *Register*, 371.

107 Cassidy-Welch, *Imprisonment*, 2–4, 15–16, 19; Guy Geltner, *The medieval prison: a social history*, Princeton, NJ 2008, 82–6.

rule or committed crimes. From as early as the eleventh century, many monasteries were equipped with their own prisons, which housed both their own members who had transgressed and criminals from the secular world outside.[108] According to Langlois, Mont-aux-Malades had a prison.[109] As *leprosarium* statutes demonstrate, anxieties about discipline and enclosure were very much at play in the regulation of these communities.[110] At all monastic communities, including leper houses, there was particular concern to enclose religious women and to ensure that they remained chaste.[111]

Mont-aux-Malades was a site for the confinement and punishment of non-leprous religious from other communities. On his visit to the Cistercian nunnery of Saint-Aubin de Gournay (département Seine-Maritime, canton Gournay-en-Bray), north-west of Rouen, on 23 July 1256, Eudes Rigaud removed the veil from Alice de Rouen and Eustacia d'Etrépagny 'on account of their fornication'.[112] The record of this visit then states that 'we sent Agnes de Pont to the *leprosarium* at Rouen, because according to rumour she conspired in the said Eustacia's fornication and even oversaw it, and because she gave Eustacia herbs to drink, in order to kill the child conceived in her, according to what is said through rumour'.[113] Although Agnes was not punished as severely as Alice and Eustacia, her implication in the crime was considered serious enough for her to be sent away from the nunnery, presumably for a limited period until she had completed her penance.[114]

While is not certain to which of Rouen's *leprosaria* Agnes was sent, on 24 December 1266 Eudes Rigaud sent another religious who had contravened monastic discipline, John Le Grand, a canon of Rouen's La Madeleine hospital, to Mont-aux-Malades. John was 'seriously defamed of incontinence', and had behaved badly at Foville and Hotot, 'living incontinently and carrying things away from the house unlawfully'.[115] Foville and Hotot-Saint-

---

108 Johnson, *Equal in monastic profession*, 202.

109 Langlois, *Histoire*, 333–5, citing 'l'ancien code pénal' of Mont-aux-Malades. I have not located this penal code, or found other evidence of the *leprosarium*'s prison.

110 See, for example, the rules of the *leprosarium* of St Mary Magdalene, Exeter, restated in the early fifteenth century: Richards, *The medieval leper*, 140–1.

111 Cassidy-Welch, *Imprisonment*, ch. i.

112 'propter earum fornicacionem': *Regestrum*, 255; *Register*, 285; Manon Six, '71 H 1–20: fonds des Bernardines de Saint-Aubin de Gournay: répertoire numérique détaillé', unpubl. inventory, ADSM, 2008, 2.

113 'Agnetem de Ponte misimus apud leprosariam Rothomagensem, quia consensit fornicacioni dicte Eustachie, et etiam procuravit, prout fama clamat, et quia dedit dicte Eustachie herbas bibere, ut interficeretur puer conceptus in dicta Eustachia, secundum quod dicitur per famam': *Regestrum*, 255; *Register*, 285; Hicks, 'Exclusion as exile', 147.

114 Hicks, 'Exclusion as exile', 151.

115 'graviter de incontinencia diffamatum; … incontinenter vivendo et res a domo illicite absportando': *Regestrum*, 563; *Register*, 645.

Sulpice were parish churches in the Pays de Caux held by La Madeleine.[116] John could have been sent to serve in these parishes; he would have been living at some distance from the 'home' community, perhaps encouraging his bad behaviour. As a punishment, 'we proclaimed that he should make purgation on account of this canonically before the next Purification of the Virgin Mary [2 February], and we ordered the prior that he should send him to Mont-aux-Malades, to stay there until the said Purification, and meanwhile he should purge himself'.[117] Purgation involved confession, reflection upon one's sins, fasting, and perhaps even flagellation, in order to fulfil the required penance and expiate one's sin. In line with the themes of early Christian writings and the practices of ascetics such as anchorites, John was to undergo purgation to improve his spiritual condition and cleanse his soul of sin.[118]

The cases of both Agnes de Pont and John Le Grand are associated with contravention of the monastic vow of chastity, as well as with the crimes of theft and attempted abortion. Since leprosy was at times associated with lasciviousness and sexual misconduct in the Middle Ages, it is possible that Agnes and John were sent to a *leprosarium* to contemplate leprosy as a punishment for sexual transgression, in order to encourage their repentance. Equally, however, it is probable that leper houses, which confined lepers for the benefit of their souls, and were located outside towns and cities, were viewed as an appropriate destination for monastic exile, enclosure and punishment. The pious example of the resident lepers may have been the most powerful reason for the fulfilment of this role by these institutions.

Pious activities and liturgical observances were central to daily life at Mont-aux-Malades, Salle-aux-Puelles and many other medieval *leprosaria*. While the care of souls was undoubtedly a major preoccupation of these communities, worship also helped to structure communal life and regulate behaviour. This survey of the diverse manifestations of piety and liturgy at Rouen's *leprosaria* has shed particular light on the material culture of these institutions, from churches and the treasures within them, to funerary monuments and archaeological remains. Church furnishings, including paintings, reliquaries, candles and altars, created the appropriate environment in which to worship. This setting, along with liturgical music and confession, was arguably highly therapeutic for the leprous residents.[119] Although the care of the soul involved enclosing lepers and keeping them separated from the world,

---

116 Dubois, 'Les Rouennais', 30, 31.

117 'nos indiximus ei purgationem propter hoc canonice faciendam infra purificationem Beate Marie subsequentem, et precepimus priori quod eum mitteret ad Montem Leprosorum, moraturum ibidem usque ad dictam purificationem, et interim se purgaret': *Regestrum*, 563; *Register*, 645–6.

118 See Geltner, *Medieval prison*, 82–6.

119 For an assessment of perceptions of the therapeutic powers of music see Christopher

as well as subject to codes of discipline, it also created an environment that benefited their psychological wellbeing, essential for those suffering from a chronic, disfiguring and ultimately fatal disease. While this reflects the medieval understanding that tending to the soul was essential to the care of the sick, the attention paid to burial and commemoration in Rouen's *leprosaria* underlines the overriding preoccupation with the soul's fate after death that coloured all pious practices in this period.

Page, 'Music and medicine in the thirteenth century', in Peregrine Horden (ed.), *Music as medicine: the history of music therapy since antiquity*, Aldershot 2000, 109–19.

Conclusion

This study has charted the impact of, and changing responses to, a distinctive disease, leprosy, in one of the major cities of medieval Western Europe. Its findings are based upon the contents of a remarkable archive, that of the *leprosarium* of Mont-aux-Malades, one of the largest and wealthiest of such institutions in medieval France. By placing Mont-aux-Malades in the context of other leper houses and sources of evidence, the findings provide the first wide-ranging study of leprosy and charity in Rouen between the central and later Middle Ages, and shed much light on practices of charity, lay piety and property ownership in and around the city. This study also helps us to understand the dynamics and complexities of medieval society during a period of great change, under the stresses of economic growth, plague and war.

Although very few medieval people actually contracted leprosy, the disease had a significant cultural impact throughout Europe. Many factors shaped the experiences of those who suffered from it, as well as responses to it. Gender and social status played a significant role, as is revealed by the history of Rouen's female leper house, Salle-aux-Puelles, while an examination of medical responses sheds new light on the medical world of Rouen and other cities. What is clear, however, is that although responses to leprosy remained diverse and complex throughout the period, with instances of compassion towards sufferers evidenced well into the sixteenth century, there was a fundamental shift in attitudes during the fourteenth century. At that point, concern increased about the spread of disease via corrupt air, and charity for lepers ceased to be highly fashionable.

Lepers: the fine line between marginality and integration

A core issue is the extent to which leprosy sufferers at Rouen were marginalised or excluded, and how this situation changed over time.[1] Here, in providing a new regional case study, this study makes a vital contribution to

---

[1] For a discussion of the issue of marginality, comparing responses to leprosy and mental disorders see Elma Brenner, 'Marginal bodies and minds: responses to leprosy and mental disorders in late medieval Normandy', in Andrew Spicer and Jane Stevens Crawshaw (eds), *The problem and place of the social margins, 1300–1800*, London forthcoming.

our understanding of medieval leprosy.[2] The positioning of Rouen's *leprosaria* outside the city, as was the case for other Western European urban centres, undoubtedly signifies the spatial marginality of the residents of these institutions, and could suggest that an impulse to distance and confine lepers helped to motivate charity for them. Nonetheless, several leper houses, particularly Mont-aux-Malades, remained in relative proximity to Rouen and well-connected by transport routes. A location within reach of the city facilitated the transportation of agricultural produce and other supplies to and from a leper house, and also offered greater protection in times of war. Furthermore, Mont-aux-Malades, and to a lesser extent Salle-aux-Puelles, retained strong links with the city through their role as a focus of charity in the twelfth and thirteenth centuries. The fact that, as the charters show, donors expected to obtain salvation by supporting the leprous, confirms that the latter were still considered to be very much part of the Christian community. In addition, through charitable gifts Mont-aux-Malades developed property interests within the city, causing citizens to transact with the leper community and thus to form connections with it.

Mont-aux-Malades, like other leper houses in France and England, achieved further economic integration through its fair that began on the feast of St Giles (1 September) each year, established by Henry II.[3] The fair of Saint-Gilles was still taking place in the eighteenth century; it was thus, for centuries, an event of local importance.[4] Patrons of the fair travelled to the *leprosarium* itself, suggesting that they were not overly concerned about the risk of contact with the leprous, in terms of either contagion or encountering people who bore the shocking physical characteristics of leprosy. Like the holy days on which lepers begged at the cathedral, the fair was thus an occasion for the temporary social integration of lepers. In both cases, integration was permitted in the context of a religious festival, which perhaps underlined the shared Christian identity of the sick and the healthy.

The marginality of lepers was both highly nuanced and flexible, to a large extent due to distinctions of social and religious status. The leprous monks of Saint-Ouen who resided at Mont-aux-Malades in the later thirteenth century, for example, were required to live at a *leprosarium* but could nonetheless freely make visits to the abbey, within the city walls, and mix with their healthy brethren.[5] At the other end of the social spectrum, the poor lepers who received leftover food from Salle-aux-Puelles in the mid-

---

[2] For other regional case studies see, for example, Bourgeois, *Lépreux et maladreries* (Pas-de-Calais region); Touati, *Maladie et societé* (diocese of Sens); and Rawcliffe, *Leprosy* (England).

[3] For leper house fairs in France see Touati, *Maladie et societé*, 533–5; for England see Rawcliffe, *Leprosy*, 314–15.

[4] Langlois, *Histoire*, 14–15.

[5] Appendix 2, no. 86.

thirteenth century were marginal in terms of their inability to enter a leper house community and benefit from the bodily and spiritual care that it offered.[6] Such divisions changed over time, since by the later fourteenth century Mont-aux-Malades had become less exclusive, catering for itinerant lepers as well as for its more traditional constituency. Above all, the question of marginality and exclusion highlights the great variation in ideas about leprosy and contagion, and also the need for a more fundamental appreciation of the complex dynamics of medieval society.

Institutional charity

The leper house emerged as a distinctive institutional form in the twelfth century, offering long-term bodily and spiritual care to the chronically sick. These institutions were very diverse, and could become significant players in local economic and religious affairs. While Mont-aux-Malades and Salle-aux-Puelles became well-established institutions and counted among Rouen's distinguished monastic houses, there were several other leper houses around the city, probably founded in the thirteenth century or later, that were very different in character. The *leprosarium* was a highly flexible type of institution, in terms of its size, the provision that it offered, and the length of its existence. Some are known to have served specific groups of Rouen parishes and to have been furnished with a chapel. Others, such as a 'lepers' cabin' at the Porte-Saint-Ouen and a community of lepers at Répainville, are only mentioned in single documentary citations, and may have been short-lived. Broadly speaking, the earliest foundations were the largest and most enduring.

Despite the modesty of some of Rouen's leper houses, collectively they comprehensively served the wider metropolitan area, being geographically located north, south, west and east of the city. While it would be misleading to suggest that, overall, urban facilities for lepers were coordinated by the ecclesiastical, royal or municipal authorities, it is clear that the arrangements made by Rouen parishes and suburban villages resulted in a ring of *leprosaria* around the city. A similar distribution of leper houses occurred at Toulouse, London and other medieval cities.[7] The involvement of parishes in the affairs of specific leper houses, as well as the implication of parochial authorities in leprosy examinations at the end of the Middle Ages, reveals the key role played by local communities in providing for the sick and disabled, a subject that requires further study in relation to Normandy and other parts of France.

---

[6] *Regestrum*, 101, 538; *Register*, 116, 615.

[7] For Toulouse see Mundy, 'Hospitals and leprosaries', 181–205; for London see Honeybourne, 'Leper hospitals', 1–64.

It is important to note that the distinction between those lepers who lived within and those who lived outside institutions was not always clear-cut. In the fourteenth and fifteenth centuries, lepers gathered at Rouen cathedral on Sundays and on other religious festivals to receive alms; these lepers numbered both the itinerant sick and the residents of smaller *leprosaria*, institutions that depended on income from begging. Mont-aux-Malades, many of whose residents were of high social and religious status, provided for the passing sick from at least the later Middle Ages and perhaps earlier. The number of wandering lepers (or itinerant people who claimed to or were believed to have leprosy) no doubt increased in the later Middle Ages in the context of considerable social upheaval, particularly during the Hundred Years' War, which helps to explain why charity was offered to them at Mont-aux-Malades and the cathedral gates. At the same time, however, the blurring of the boundary between residence in a *leprosarium* and itinerancy suggests that, by this time, lepers had more freedom of movement in mainstream society than has hitherto been appreciated. Also by this time, Mont-aux-Malades and other *leprosaria* had more flexible residency requirements. The manner in which these phenomena played out at Rouen sheds light on attitudes towards the vagrant poor at the end of the Middle Ages, and on how practices of charity changed at this time.

Charity and identity

Although the intensity of the charity exhibited towards lepers between 1100 and 1300 was not sustained in subsequent centuries, charity occupied a prominent position in society and religious culture throughout the central and later Middle Ages. The generosity of the laity was crucial to the support of Rouen's *leprosaria*, from the twelfth-century charity of the Anglo-Norman royal family onwards.[8] Broadly speaking, charity operated on two different planes: within leper houses, hospitals and monasteries lay staff and the religious tended the sick and poor; beyond the walls of these institutions, benefactors supported these activities by making donations of money, land, property and objects. These donations were made in perpetuity, since donors envisaged a continuation of the worldly *status quo* that aligned with the eternity of the spiritual realm towards which their charitable endeavours were directed. Works of charity were one aspect of a web of devotional practices, including the commemoration of souls, the veneration of saints and their relics, and the lighting of sacred spaces. Charity was also practised by confraternities and guilds, as well as within the context of the parish; it is

---

[8] On the role of the laity in charity from the twelfth century see Brodman, *Charity and religion*, 178–9.

hoped that the findings presented here will illuminate further research into the charitable activities of these bodies, in Rouen and other cities.[9]

Charity was reciprocal, offering benefits to donors as well as to the people whom they assisted. While benefactors accrued spiritual merit through their good works, these works also played a significant role in affirming their social and religious identity. For the Augustinian canons of Mont-aux-Malades, assisting lepers was a key aspect of fulfilling their religious vocation. For the numerous burgesses of Rouen who made donations to the leper house in the thirteenth century, charity was a means of displaying their piety and good character to their peers, with whom good social and business relationships were essential. The summaries of the burgesses's charters provided in appendix 2 shed light on the broader social context for the creation of these documents. Particularly in the first decades of the thirteenth century, a number of acts were confirmed by the mayor of Rouen; occasionally, the seal of the communal government was added.[10] As well as evidencing bureaucratic practice at this time, the intervention of the mayor and commune reveals that, by witnessing charters, multiple members of the urban elite were implicated in the practice of charity.

For a smaller number of lay people, namely those who entered Mont-aux-Malades and Salle-aux-Puelles as lay brethren, charity had more radical implications, marking the transformation of their identity as they began to live alongside lepers and to care for them. While both men and women took this step, the bodily care of the sick was a particularly female preoccupation in this period. Women's role is reflected by the high number of lay sisters at Mont-aux-Malades recorded in the *Register* of Eudes Rigaud, as well as by the many names of hospital sisters listed in the fifteenth-century memorial book of La Madeleine hospital.[11] Elsewhere in France, communities of Cistercian nuns took on the administration of *leprosaria* in the thirteenth century, revealing that the needs of lepers offered practical and spiritual opportunities to religious women.[12] There were both similarities and differences among men and women in terms of piety and charity, engagement in medical practice and access to care when they themselves became sick. In particular, the fact that Salle-aux-Puelles, unlike Mont-aux-Malades, discriminated according to gender testifies to the varied arrangements made for lepers in this period, even though in all leper communities the sexes were segregated.

[9] For an overview of the charity provided by confraternities and parishes see ibid. 187–221. On confraternities in medieval Normandy see Catherine Vincent, *Des Charités bien ordonnées: les confréries normandes de la fin du XIIIe siècle au début du XVIe siècle*, Paris 1988.

[10] See, for example, appendix 2, nos 10, 22.

[11] *Regestrum*, 325, 513; *Register*, 371, 585; BM, Rouen, MS Y42.

[12] Some Cistercian nunneries also developed from communities of women who were already tending the sick: Lester, *Creating Cistercian nuns*, 118–19, 129–34.

Rouen, Upper Normandy and France

By examining leprosy and charity in a specific locality, the city of Rouen and its surroundings, this book adds a study of an important region of medieval France to the scholarship in this field. Upper Normandy was a strategically vital area, affording access to the River Seine and the sea, and was a zone of great agricultural fertility. Since Rouen's leper houses had semi-rural locations, and some had significant rural estates, the history of these institutions illuminates many aspects of the wider history of Upper Normandy, particularly in terms of the landholding and agricultural activities of monastic communities.

Yet, above all, the study of leprosy and charity in Rouen contributes to our understanding of medieval cities, in France and other parts of Europe, given its major importance in the central and later Middle Ages. Consideration of responses to leprosy in Rouen sheds light on not only urban welfare provision and medical practice, but also on the city's religious culture and social networks: for example, the significance of the parish as a social and administrative unit and the prominence of the city's merchants, as well as the presence and identities of a range of medical practitioners in and around Rouen, particularly physicians and surgeons. A broad chronology, spanning the twelfth to fifteenth centuries, reveals both major changes in the city and striking continuities, such as the entrenched dominance of the major monastic houses.

As a recently published work on medicine and health in late medieval Montpellier demonstrates, the investigation of the medical history of a medieval city can greatly enhance our understanding of the broader dynamics of urban society.[13] Achieving such wider insights has been a core aim here, establishing key lines of enquiry which it is hoped will continue to be pursued by researchers in the future. Indeed, more remains to be discovered from medieval Rouen's rich written and material heritage about society, religion and responses to disease in the Middle Ages.

---

[13] Geneviève Dumas, *Santé et société à Montpellier à la fin du moyen âge*, Leiden 2015.

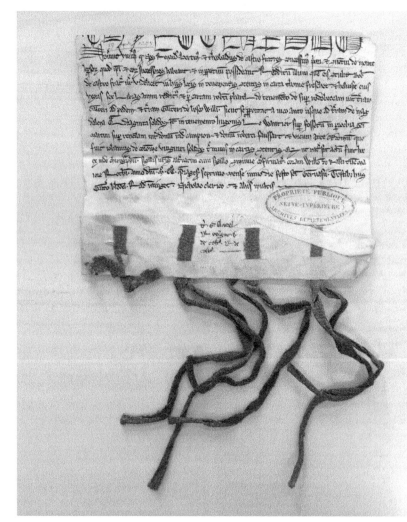

Figure 10. Charter of Renaud, Bertin and Theobald du Châtel, brothers, granting the transfer of a rent to the leper house of Mont-aux-Malades by their brother Robin du Châtel, 19 June 1247. ADSM, Rouen, 25HP1(8).

APPENDIX 1

A Note on Sources

Most of the documentary evidence for leprosy in medieval Rouen relates to the leper houses of Mont-aux-Malades and Salle-aux-Puelles, since these were religious institutions that retained their own records, particularly deeds of property, and left their trace in other documents, such as the *Register* of Eudes Rigaud. A much larger body of material survives for Mont-aux-Malades than for Salle-aux-Puelles. The former has an unusually rich and well-preserved archive, held at the Archives départementales de Seine-Maritime, Rouen.[1] It consists of at least three hundred medieval charters (*see* Figure 10 for an example dated 19 June 1247), as well as other documents from the sixteenth to the eighteenth centuries. The twelfth- and thirteenth-century charters are in Latin; from the end of the thirteenth century the documents are increasingly written in French. The great majority of the charters mark donations and sales of Rouen property to Mont-aux-Malades by the city's burgesses in the thirteenth century. Many are confirmed by Rouen's mayors, reflecting the social circles within which the burgesses moved, and making it possible to give an approximate date to undated documents.[2] Mont-aux-Malades' rededication to St Thomas Becket in about 1174 also makes it possible to date charters that refer to this dedication to about 1174 or later.

Other relevant manuscripts are housed in the ADSM, the Bibliothèque municipale, Rouen,[3] the Archives nationales, Paris and the British Library, London. The ecclesiastical archives in the ADSM (Série G) contain records of the examination of suspected lepers in the sixteenth century. The BM, Rouen, houses the fifteenth-century memorial book of La Madeleine hospital (MS Y42), which sheds light on the unification of Salle-aux-Puelles with La Madeleine in 1366, and on patterns of charitable benefaction at Rouen.

There is no extant cartulary for Mont-aux-Malades or Salle-aux-Puelles, although cartularies survive for several other French *leprosaria*.[4] However,

---

[1] ADSM, deposit 25HP.

[2] Mayoral periods of office are listed in Farin, *Histoire*, ii. 102–3; Chéruel, *Histoire*, i. 359–73; Mollat, *Histoire de Rouen*, 427–8; and Six, 'The burgesses of Rouen', 273.

[3] In the course of work on this book the medieval municipal archives of Rouen were transferred from the BM to the ADSM. Since I consulted this deposit at the BM, I have retained the BM location descriptions (for example, 'Chartrier de la ville, Tiroir 324'), but readers should be alerted to the relocation of this material.

[4] See, for example, *Cartulaire de la léproserie*; Mesmin, 'The leper hospital of Saint Gilles de Pont-Audemer'; Tabuteau, 'Une Léproserie normande'; and *Recueil d'actes de Saint-Lazare*.

for Mont-aux-Malades the conservation of a large number of charters, many of which bear a label or shelf mark, is indicative of careful record-keeping and a high level of administrative organisation. No books or mentions of books survive for either institution, although both presumably owned books. One set of rules was issued for Mont-aux-Malades by Peter de Collemezzo, archbishop of Rouen in May 1237; twelve years later (August 1249), Eudes Rigaud drew up statutes for Salle-aux-Puelles.[5]

The visitation records of Eudes Rigaud, compiled between 1248 and 1269, are an important source of information about both these leper house communities in the mid-thirteenth century.[6] The *Register* records the archbishop's numerous visits to parish churches, monasteries, hospitals and *leprosaria* in the archdiocese of Rouen. Unlike in England, where a bishop could only visit hospitals and *leprosaria* by right of patronage (not by episcopal right), it is clear that Rouen's archbishop could freely visit many hospitals and *leprosaria*.[7] Although the *Register* is an exceptionally rich source of information about religious life in thirteenth-century Normandy, it does need to be handled with care. The archbishop and his entourage were searching for problems and transgressions that required correction, meaning that they are probably more likely to have recorded their negative findings than the non-problematic situations they encountered.[8] Nonetheless, useful comparisons can be drawn between the different religious communities documented in the *Register*, which suggest that both Mont-aux-Malades and Salle-aux-Puelles were well-administered and in a relatively good financial state at this time.

Correspondence relating to the dispute between Thomas Becket and Henry II in the second half of the twelfth century also sheds light on Mont-aux-Malades. Nicholas, the leper house's first known prior, was a close friend of Becket's, and the two men exchanged several letters in the 1160s during the archbishop's exile from England (1164–70).[9] These letters reveal that Nicholas moved in courtly circles: in late 1164 he recounted his meetings on Becket's behalf with the Empress Matilda and Arnulf, bishop of Lisieux (1141–81), and he kept the exiled archbishop informed regarding Henry II's

---

[5]   AN, Paris, S4889B, dossier 13, doc. (xxi), fos 1r–2r (Mont-aux-Malades rules); *Regestrum*, 101–2; *Register*, 115–17 (Salle-aux-Puelles statutes).

[6]   *Regestrum*; *Register*. Élisabeth Lalou and Alexis Grélois at the University of Rouen are currently preparing a new digital edition of the *Register* (Bibliothèque nationale, Paris, MS Latin 1245). Although I have consulted the published English translation of the text (*Register*), the translations in this book are my own, since the published translation has occasional errors.

[7]   On episcopal visitation of hospitals in England see Watson, 'Fundatio, ordinatio and statuta, 54–62.

[8]   See Hicks, *Religious life*, 11, and Davis, *Holy bureaucrat*, 1.

[9]   For Thomas Becket's correspondence see *Materials for the history of Thomas Becket, archbishop of Canterbury*, ed. J. C. Robertson (Rolls Series, 1875–85), v–vii, and CTB.

movements.[10] One letter, ostensibly addressed by Becket to Nicholas after 12 June 1166, was almost certainly written by John of Salisbury, who wrote two further letters to Prior Nicholas in his own name in late 1166 and between December 1167 and March 1168.[11]

Finally, there is important material evidence for leprosy and charity in medieval Rouen. On the site of Mont-aux-Malades, the remains of the twelfth-century church of Saint-Jacques are still standing, while the late twelfth- and thirteenth-century fabric of the church of Saint-Thomas is incorporated in a structure heavily restored in the nineteenth century, that functions as a parish church today. Inside this church, the medieval tombstone of Matilda, wife of Laurence Chamberlain (d. 1293) survives, testifying to the burial of a charitable patron at Mont-aux-Malades. At Petit-Quevilly, the chapel of Saint-Julien that served Salle-aux-Puelles remains, and contains the twelfth-century wall paintings of the Infancy of Christ that were commissioned for it in the third quarter of the twelfth century when it was a royal chapel. Although no archaeological work has been conducted on the sites of Rouen's *leprosaria* since the nineteenth century, recent excavations elsewhere in Normandy and in England, particularly on the site of Saint-Thomas at Aizier (between Rouen and Le Havre) and at St Mary Magdalen, Winchester, provide important contextual data regarding the prevalence of leprosy in, and the built environment of, leper houses.[12]

[10] Nicholas to Becket, Christmas season, 1164, *CTB* i. 158–69 (no. 41), and August 1167, 622–3 (no. 132).

[11] Becket/John of Salisbury to Nicholas, after 12 June 1166, ibid. i. 342–7 (no. 83); Becket/John of Salisbury to Nicholas, here dated 'probably early 1166', John of Salisbury to Nicholas, 'probably about the end of 1166', and c. Dec. 1167–Mar. 1168, in *The letters of John of Salisbury*, ii. 64–7 (no. 157), 250–3 (no. 188), 452–7 (no. 239).

[12] On Aizier see Niel and Truc, 'La Chapelle Saint-Thomas d'Aizier', http://w3.unicaen.fr/ufr/histoire/craham/spip.php?article120&lang=fr (accessed 24 June 2013); on Winchester see Roffey, 'Medieval leper hospitals', 206–7, 210–11, 221, 222, 225–7.

APPENDIX 2

Charters and Other Documents Relating to Leprosy: Mont-aux-Malades, Salle-aux-Puelles and Other Communities of Lepers in Rouen, c. 1100–c. 1500

Since this summary list consists mainly of charters, with a smaller number of testaments, papal bulls and other types of document, it is organised according to the names of the key protagonists in the texts, who are listed alphabetically by their Christian names. Unless otherwise stated, the original documents are in Latin. The smaller number that are written in French, from the late thirteenth century onwards, are indicated. While protagonists' Christian names are anglicised to Andrew, Matilda, James and so on, surnames appear in either their modern French form (e.g. Nicholas de la Commune) or, when a French equivalent for a Latin word could not be found, in the original Latin (e.g. Walter and Robert Goobondi). Each entry provides a summary of the key points within a document, rather than a full translation (or in all cases a full summary). The reference at the foot of each entry denotes the document's location in the Archives départementales de Seine-Maritime, Rouen, the Archives nationales, Paris, or another repository. The majority of the documents are located in the Mont-aux-Malades archive, deposit 25HP in the ADSM, and are referenced as precisely as possible. For example, no. 9 (25HP47(11)(xxii)) is document (xxii) in folder 11 of box 25HP47. I have supplied the folder and document numbers; the box numbers are those ascribed by the ADSM. Since I undertook my research at the ADSM, the material within some boxes has been rearranged. However, my references should still make it possible for an individual document to be located easily within a box. Where relevant, entries also mention publications that provide editions or citations of documents.

1. Adam Rigaud (de Verneau), dean of Rouen, and the chapter of Rouen cathedral

1297 (original)

The dean and chapter of Rouen give notice that William de Flavacourt, archbishop of Rouen (1275–1306) has granted that Mont-aux-Malades should enjoy the revenues of the church of Saint-Aignan.

[ADSM, 25HP1(4)(iv)]

2. Agnes, wife of Ralph Le Comte, of the parish of Saint-Patrice, Rouen

April 1262 (original charter of the official of Rouen, giving notice of Agnes's gifts)

With the consent of her husband Ralph, for the salvation of her soul and the souls of her ancestors, Agnes has donated in pure and perpetual alms to Mont-aux-Malades a house in the parish of Saint-Patrice, Rouen, two pieces of land in the parish of Saint-Godard, Rouen, and other gifts.

[ADSM, 25HP3(6)(ii)]

3. Alan Brito, canon of Rouen cathedral, Adam, almoner of La Trinité-du-Mont, Rouen, and Matthew Faber, cleric

July 1227 (two original charters)

Alan, Adam and Matthew resolve a dispute between Roger de Bonneville and his brother Lucas, clerics, and Mont-aux-Malades regarding a tenement in the parish of Saint-Martin-sur-Renelle, Rouen. They establish that Roger and Lucas and their heirs will hold the tenement, paying 25 *sous* annual rent to Mont-aux-Malades. In return for this rent, the prior and brothers of Mont-aux-Malades will exercise their right of justice with regard to the tenement.

[ADSM, 25HP1(8)(i), (iv)]

4. Alexander III, pope (1159–81)

n.d. (c. 1174–81; original and two seventeenth-century copies)

Alexander gives greetings to the prior and canons of Mont-aux-Malades who are responsible for the care of lepers. He recognises their great burden, both in serving God and in caring for lepers and the poor. Following their requests, he confirms their possession of the church of Saint-Sauveur at Nointot and their mill at Maromme.

[ADSM, 25HP7(v) (original), 25HP46(2)(iv) (seventeenth-century copy), AN, Paris, S4889B, dossier 13 (seventeenth-century copy); edited in Langlois, *Histoire*, 425–60]

5. Alide d'Espiney, widow

1252 (original and seventeenth-century copy)

For the salvation of herself, her parents and all her ancestors, Alide has donated to Mont-aux-Malades 4 *sous* of Tours annual rent due from the tenement of Roscelin Thibart (Huguelou), situated at the head of the rue Courière in front of the stone cross. Her charter is witnessed by John (de Beuzevillette), prior of Mont-aux-Malades, Henry, *bailli* of Mont-aux-Malades, William Muchart, John Faber and Richard de Baiocis, canons of Mont-aux-Malades, and Brother William de Bretteville.

[AN, Paris, S4889B, dossier 13, nos 19 (seventeenth-century copy), 20 (original)]

6. Alix, daughter of Osbert de Préaux, widow of John de Hodenc

n.d. (c. 1174–1200; original), at Rouen cathedral

With the consent of her eldest son Giles, Alix has donated a piece of land at Saint-Gervais, Rouen (which she held through marriage) to three religious houses: the abbey of Sainte-Marie de Beaubec (which the gift favours), Mont-aux-Malades and La Madeleine hospital, Rouen. Her gift is made for the salvation of herself and her husband, ancestors, successors and friends. The land returns annually 13 *livres* of Anjou. Annually on the feast of St Remigius, 100 *sous* are to be paid to the monks of Beaubec, 4 *livres* to Mont-aux-Malades, and 4 *livres* to La Madeleine hospital. Her husband John de Hodenc made this gift during his life, and she now confirms it after his death.

[ADSM, 25HP1(10); Langlois, *Histoire*, 93]

7. Andrew de Beuzemouchel (Bernières)

(a) n.d. (c. 1174–84: notification by Rotrou of Warwick, archbishop of Rouen [1165–84], in an original *vidimus* of the *vicomte* of Caudebec, 1384)

Andrew donates to Mont-aux-Malades in perpetual alms his men at Nointot (nine names are listed) and the whole tenement that they hold from him there.

[ADSM, 25HP3(2)(iii); Langlois, *Histoire*, 87–8]

(b) n.d. (c. 1174–1200; original)

For the salvation of his soul and those of his ancestors, Andrew has donated a rent to God and Mont-aux-Malades 'and the poor of Christ [there] labouring too much in their infirmity' when departing on a remote pilgrimage.

[ADSM, 25HP47(13)]

8. Andrew, son of Robert de Fécamp and Hendeborge de Torella

November 1217 (original)

Andrew grants 4 *livres*, 3 *sous*, 3 *deniers* and 1 capon of rent to Mont-aux-Malades due from lands in the parishes of Saint-Martin-sur-Renelle and Saint-Hilaire, Rouen. In return, he is to receive 2 bushels of corn and 4 ounces of pepper annually. He also receives 40 *livres* in recognition of his grant.

[ADSM, 25HP1(8)(xxviii)]

9. The *bailli* of Gisors

1296 (original, in French), at Lyons

The *bailli* of Gisors resolves a dispute between Richard, prior of Mont-aux-Malades (prior until 1298) and James de Lyons, the official in charge of collecting pannage (the due paid to the lord of a forest for the right to graze pigs there) in the forest of Lyons. James de Lyons has claimed a forfeit of sixty-five pigs from Prior Richard. The prior denies the forfeit; James maintains that he seized the pigs because Richard had not brought evidence of Mont-aux-Malades's right to exemption from paying pannage to an appeal case. Richard argues that he had previously shown such evidence to the master in charge of pannage, and had not therefore been required to bring it to this appeal. The *bailli* of Gisors rules in Prior Richard's favour, instructing that he should take the pigs back.

[ADSM, 25HP47(11)(xxii)]

10. Bartholomew, Matthew and Roger, sons of Bartholomew Bataille

n.d. (1198 or 1202: confirmed by Ralph de Cailli, mayor of Rouen, who added the seal of the commune; original)

For the salvation of their souls and those of their parents, ancestors and successors, Bartholomew, Matthew and Roger have given to God and the church of Saint-Thomas of Mont-aux-Malades, in free and perpetual alms, the 10 *sous* of rent which their brother Geoffrey Bataille returned to them annually from the house which he held from them in the district of Saint-Martin, Rouen.

[ASDM, 25HP1. On the leading Rouen burgess Bartholomew Bataille and his sons see Six, 'The burgesses of Rouen', 265.]

11. ?Bartholomew, prior and the chapter of Mont-aux-Malades

October 1237 (original, with the seal of Mont-aux-Malades attached)

The prior and chapter of Mont-aux-Malades acknowledge the gift by the dean and chapter of Rouen cathedral of the right to take two loaves daily from the celebration of mass at the cathedral. The prior and chapter of Mont-aux-Malades, and their successors, pledge that they will only claim this gift by the dean and chapter's will, and only for so long as it pleases the dean and chapter.

[ASDM, 25HP10; Langlois, *Histoire*, 116]

12. Cecily Talbot, dowager countess of Hereford (d. 1207)

n.d. (c. 1173–4; a charter of Gilbert Foliot, bishop of London [1163–87])

Gilbert Foliot gives notice that he has granted the church of Vange (Essex, diocese of London) to Mont-aux-Malades in perpetual alms. He does this with the consent of Lady Cecily Talbot, in whose patrimony the church of Vange is situated. He has also appointed Prior Herbert of Mont-aux-Malades to the church of Vange. He strengthens his charter by attaching his seal and those of Cecily Talbot and 'St Thomas, a short time previously archbishop of Canterbury'.

[Edited in Langlois, *Histoire*, 423–4; *The letters and charters of Gilbert Foliot*, 472 (no. 436). See Langlois, *Histoire*, 81, and I. J. Sanders, *English baronies: a study of their origin and descent, 1086–1327*, Oxford 1960, 144.]

13. Charles v, king of France (1364–80)

(a) 31 August 1366 (in the fifteenth-century memorial book of Rouen's La Madeleine hospital)

On this day King Charles donated to La Madeleine the church of Saint-Julien of Salle-aux-Puelles, formerly called Sainte-Marie of Quevilly, with all its rights and possessions. In return, the community of La Madeleine must celebrate in perpetuity in the church of Saint-Julien a Mass every Sunday and on solemn days and feasts. It must also celebrate in the church of La Madeleine, daily at the altar of St Eustache before the image of the king, a Mass of the Holy Spirit while he is alive, and a Mass of the Dead after his death. This will be called the 'Mass of the king'. Every day after compline, when the brothers are assembled in the sick ward, the priest who has sung compline should exhort the paupers lying there to pray for the king and all the church's benefactors. The king has also donated to La Madeleine some sacerdotal vestments, a gilt chalice with a 'baiser de paix', and two gilt flasks. He has also bequeathed 300 *livres* of Tours in gold Francs.

[BM, Rouen, MS Y42, fo. 50v; also fo. 54r (death of Charles v, 1380). See also Duchemin, *Petit-Quevilly*, 233, and Dubois, 'Les Rouennais face à la mort', 83–5.]

(b) November 1366 (original and *vidimus* of the official of Rouen, 1366, and ?seventeenth-century printed copy), at Rouen

The king gives notice that he has donated in perpetuity to the prior of La Madeleine the patronage of the church of Saint-Julien and the house of Salle-aux-Puelles in the forest of Rouvray near Rouen, with all their appendages and rights. The prior of La Madeleine accepts these in his name and those of the brothers, prioress and sisters of La Madeleine. King Charles hopes that the care of the souls of the miserable persons infected with leprosy at Salle-aux-Puelles will henceforth be exercised more devotedly and more thoughtfully, that the religious will administer to these persons a sufficiency of victuals, and that those secular priests who previously had charge of the church of Saint-Julien will continue to serve in it. He asks the archbishop of Rouen to ensure that the church of Saint-Julien is unified, annexed and ceded to La Madeleine in such a way that, when the rector, curate or administrator currently serving the church of Saint-Julien retires, dies or otherwise abandons his post, the prior of La Madeleine will take corporal possession of the church with all rights and appendages, and convert them to the use of the brothers and sisters of La Madeleine. Nonetheless, the care of souls in the church and in Salle-aux-Puelles should continue to be exercised, divine office should be celebrated there, and the sacraments should be administered, as is the custom there at present. Temporal affairs at Salle-aux-Puelles should be administered in a praiseworthy manner, lest there should be a lacking of humanity and temporality to the miserable persons residing there, now and in the future. A sufficiency of temporals should be administered to every single one of these persons, so that they should not have need of victuals or have to collect timber. The prior and brothers are to celebrate regular masses on the king's behalf in La Madeleine's church, and are to commend him to their special memory; the prioress and the sisters, and the paupers received in the hospital, are to [perform] devoted and continual prayers, intercessions and orations on his behalf.

[ADSM, 27HP95 (original and *vidimus* of Thomas Baudri, official of Rouen);

ADSM, H-Dépôt 1, A39 (?seventeenth-century printed copy). See also Duchemin, *Petit-Quevilly*, 232–4, and René Herval, *Histoire de Rouen*, Rouen 1947–9, i. 149.]

14. The dean (unnamed) of the church of Saint-Cande-le-Vieux, Rouen

January 1266 (original)

The dean of Saint-Cande-le-Vieux gives notice that the treasurers of the church of Sotteville-lès-Rouen have taken in perpetual fief and hereditary possession from Mont-aux-Malades 'a certain leper house … or piece of land' in the parish of Sotteville-lès-Rouen, for 5 *sous* annual rent. The rent is to be returned to the dean of Saint-Cande-le-Vieux and his brothers 'by the said treasurers and their successors or the lepers who in time will be there'. The religious of Mont-aux-Malades are held to the agreement that, in exchange for the said rent, the said fief or piece of land is granted in alms by them for the construction of the said leper house.

[ADSM, 25HP1(16)(ii); edited in Tabuteau, 'Léproseries', 178. See also Deschamps, 'Léproseries', 31–2; P. Duchemin, *Sotteville-lès-Rouen, et le faubourg de Saint-Sever*, Rouen 1893, repr. Paris 1990, 20–1. The church of Sotteville-lès-Rouen came under the patronage of Saint-Cande-le-Vieux, a collegiate church: Lemoine and Tanguy, *Rouen*, 36–7.]

15. Elias Sobet and his wife Peronelle, of the parish of Saint-Maclou, Rouen

1292 (the Monday before Ash Wednesday) (original act, in French, of the *vicomte* of Rouen)

Elias and Peronelle have taken in fief and perpetual hereditary possession, from the abbey of Sainte-Catherine (La Trinité-du-Mont, Rouen) and Mont-aux-Malades, a vacant plot of land in Saint-Maclou parish, for 32 *sous* (current money) annual rent to be shared equally between the two religious houses.

(An earlier donation of land had evidently jointly favoured Mont-aux-Malades and La Trinité-du-Mont; each house had the same stake in the land.)

[ADSM, 25HP6]

16. Emmeline Karite, widow

July 1221 (original act of Roger, dean and the chapter of Rouen cathedral)

Emmeline has sold 15 *deniers* of annual rent due from a tenement to Mont-aux-Malades, in return for 12 *sous* of Tours.

[ADSM, 25HP36]

17. Erembourg de Ponce Liatons, her son Robert, and Geoffrey Parent, of the parish of Saint-Maclou, Rouen

1265 (original act of the official of Rouen)

Erembourg, Robert and Geoffrey have granted to Mont-aux-Malades any rights they held to a piece of land in Saint-Maclou parish.

[ADSM, 25HP6]

18. Erembourg de Tancarville, widow of Robert de Tancarville

February 1234 (original, confirmed before Geoffrey du Val-Richer, mayor of Rouen; also an original confirmation by the official of Rouen, dated January 1234)

For 9 *sous* of Tours (15 *sous* of Tours in the act of the official of Rouen), Erembourg has sold to Prior Ralph de Longueville and the community of Mont-aux-Malades 12 *deniers* (usual money at Rouen) annual rent which William Angevin paid her from his tenement in the rue *Caprario*. The tenement is situated between the land of La Madeleine hospital and that of William Angevin, in the fief of Mont-aux-Malades.

(The Tancarville family were hereditary chamberlains of Normandy and were among 'those families, mostly of secondary rank before 1204' whose importance in the duchy increased after 1204: Thompson, 'L'Aristocratie anglo-normande', 182; Power, *The Norman frontier*, 450.)

[ADSM, 25HP1(23)(ii) (charter of Erembourg de Tancarville); 25HP6 (charter of the official of Rouen)]

19. Eudes Rigaud, archbishop of Rouen (1248–75)

(a) October 1248: a bull of Pope Innocent IV (1243–54) (original)

Innocent IV gives notice that the archbishop of Rouen [Eudes Rigaud] intends to grant a piece of land to the lepers of Aliermont, for a house to be built there for them. He plans to found a church there in his *villa*, and wishes it to have land for a cemetery, and a small lodging for a priest.

[ADSM, G1123(ix)]

(b) 1253, at Déville (original)

Eudes Rigaud resolves a dispute between Nicholas, rector of the church of Bois-Guillaume and the prior and community of Mont-aux-Malades, regarding revenues which Mont-aux-Malades collects in the fief of Bois-Guillaume.

[ADSM, 25HP1(2)(ii)]

20. Florent de Grémonville, knight

n.d. (1176, 1177, 1179, 1180, 1182 or 1190 [from c. 1174]; accompanying charter of William de Malpalu is witnessed by Bartholomew Fergant as mayor of Rouen, in an original *vidimus* of the *vicomte* of Rouen, 1301)

Florent confirms his gift in pure and perpetual alms to Mont-aux-Malades of the rent of 13 *sous* (current money) which he enjoyed from the land of Mont-de-la-Coudre and its two hosts, all of which William de Malpalu held from him.

[ADSM, 25HP1(2)(i); Langlois, *Histoire*, 87]

21. Geoffrey, count of Anjou (1129–51), duke of Normandy (1145–50)

(a) n.d. (1145–50) (original and two seventeenth-century copies), at Rouen

Geoffrey of Anjou orders the *vicomte* of Rouen to deliver 40 *sous* of Rouen each month to the lepers of Rouen, in accordance with the gift of King Henry [Henry I, king of England (1100–35) and duke of Normandy (1106–35)], as is confirmed in his charter.

[AN, Paris, *K23 nos 15 22 (original), 15 22b (*vidimus* issued by the *vicomté* of Rouen, 28 Dec. 1437); ADSM, 25HP46 (seventeenth-century copy); 25HP54(2), fo. 1r (late seventeenth-century [from 1674] copy). Edited in Langlois, *Histoire*, 397; *Recueil des actes*, introduction, 136; Charles Homer Haskins, *Norman institutions*, Cambridge, MA 1918, 142 (and plate 7a); *Regesta* iii. 269 (no. 730). See also Haskins, *Norman institutions*, 134, 151.]

(b) n.d. (1145–50, in a confirmation dated May 1259 by John de Beuzevil-lette, prior of Mont-aux-Malades, in a seventeenth-century copy)

Geoffrey of Anjou gives notice to all the ministers of the church, and all the faithful, that Nicholas, prior of Mont-aux-Malades, and the whole community of canons and poor lepers there, have taken the brothers and sisters of the fraternity of the palmers of Rouen into their fraternity.

[ADSM, 25HP46 (seventeenth-century copy). See also Langlois, *Histoire*, 3–4, and Haskins, *Norman institutions*, 134.]

22. Geoffrey, son of Bartholomew Bataille

n.d. (1198 or 1202: confirmed by Ralph de Cailli, mayor of Rouen, who added the seal of the commune; original)

For the salvation of his soul and those of his parents, ancestors and successors, Geoffrey has given to God and the church of Saint-Thomas of Mont-aux-Malades, and the brothers healthy and sick serving God there, a *masura* of land [a house] in the district of Saint-Martin, Rouen, situated between the church of Saint-Martin and the house of Enard Village. His father Bartholomew Bataille gave him this house as [part of] his portion of inheritance.

[ADSM, 25HP1]

23. Geoffrey de Carville, knight

February 1240 (in an original *vidimus* of the *vicomte* of Rouen, 1293)

Geoffrey has donated to Mont-aux-Malades 33 *sous*, 6 capons of annual rent, due from tenements at Carville, in front of the church of Saint-Pierre, and Répainville.

[ADSM, 25HP1(8)(xviii); Langlois, *Histoire*, 93–4. Mont-aux-Malades held the church of Saint-Pierre of Carville as a gift from Ralph, son of Stephen in February 1161.]

24. Geoffrey II, dean, and the chapter of Rouen cathedral

n.d. (c. 1154–74, probably c. 1160; original)

Dean Geoffrey II and the chapter of Rouen cathedral confirm the purchase by Mont-aux-Malades of a mill at Maromme from Macharius and his heirs, for 15 marks of silver. Annually on the feast of St Remigius, Mont-aux-Malades is to pay 3 *sous* rent for the mill to the dean and chapter. This 'public sale' ('emptio publice') was cele-brated in the presence of the dean and chapter and seven royal justices, including Renaud de Saint-Valéry, Roscelin, son of Clarembaud and William de Malpalu.

[AN, Paris, S4889B, liasse 1 no. 6; edited in Haskins, *Norman institutions*, 325–6. See also Langlois, *Histoire*, 16.]

25. Geoffrey Glosseboc

n.d. (c. 1174–90; witnessed by Bartholomew Fergant as mayor of Rouen; original)

Geoffrey has granted the sale of land and a house in the parish of Saint-André, Rouen to Mont-aux-Malades by Renaud de Saint-[Valéry] [the second part of Renaud's surname is indecipherable, but he may well be synonymous with Henry II's justice, Renaud de Saint-Valéry].

[ADSM, 25HP1(1)(iii)]

26. Geoffrey Le Cras, of the parish of Pîtres (Eure, canton Pont-de-l'Arche)

16 August 1302 (in a *vidimus* of the official of Rouen, 12 Sept. 1304. Offi-cial's preamble in Latin; Geoffrey's text in French)

Geoffrey's testament. He was in service to the abbess and community of Saint-Amand, Rouen, for more than thirty years, until he became sick and lost his sight. Recognising how much he had depended on Saint-Amand, he previously donated all his property to the community, excepting 40 *livres* of Tours, which he retained to give to whomsoever he wished. His bequests benefit individuals, religious communi-ties and needy groups. Among the latter two categories are a bequest of 20 *sous* to Rouen cathedral; 60 *sous* to the church at Pîtres (Notre-Dame), his parish, with a rent of 20 *sous* towards the lighting of the church; 20 *sous* to Rouen's La Madeleine hospital; 20 *sous* to Mont-aux-Malades; 5 *sous* to the hospital of the Porte-Saint-Ouen, Rouen; 3 *sous* to the leper house of Pont-de-l'Arche; 3 *sous* each to the leper house of Pont-Saint-Pierre, the house of Sainte-Marguerite of Val-de-Reuil, and the leper house of Chant d'Oisel; 20 *sous* to the poor women of Pîtres; 40 *sous* to the church of Lire; 60 *sous* to the poor women of Lire.

[Edited in Marie-Josèphe Le Cacheux, *Histoire de l'abbaye de Saint-Amand de Rouen, des origines à la fin du XVIe siècle*, Caen 1937, 263–5, in which it is stated at p. 264 n. 1 that the act by which Geoffrey Le Cras donated all his property to Saint-Amand dates from 13 May 1293. For the leper house of Pont-de-l'Arche see AN, Paris, S4890A, dossier 4 (document of 19 June 1674).]

27. Geoffrey Pèlerin of the parish of Saint-Martin-sur-Renelle, Rouen and John Beaunies of the parish of Saint-Ouen, Rouen

September 1237 (original, issued by the official of Rouen)

In return for 20 *sous* of Tours, Geoffrey and John have given up to Mont-aux-Malades all rights and hereditary claims they held to a property in Saint-Martin-sur-Renelle parish [this property was donated by William and Alicia Le Tort Bouglarius in September 1233].

[ADSM, 25HP1(8)(xxv)]

28. Giles, son of Stephen, son of Tehard

n.d. (1195 or 1198–1200; witnessed by Matthew Le Gros as mayor of Rouen; original)

Giles has donated 60 *sous* of rent to Mont-aux-Malades in perpetual alms, due from his house in the parish of Saint-Vincent, Rouen, and his fief in the district of Estopée. The gift is made for the salvation of his soul and those of his father, mother and all his ancestors, 'and especially for the soul of my brother Nicholas, as he set out in his testament and I agreed with him'.

[ADSM, 25HP1(18)(i)]

29. Gregory XI, pope (1370–8)

Eleventh calends of July 1377 (original, *vidimus* and ?eighteenth-century copy), at Villeneuve

Pope Gregory gives greetings to the bishop of Paris. He recently saw the petition of the prior, brothers, prioress and sisters of La Madeleine hospital, Rouen, regarding King Charles's gift of the parish church of Saint-Julien and the house of Salle-aux-Puelles to La Madeleine. Gregory orders the bishop of Paris to annex and unify Salle-aux-Puelles and the church of Saint-Julien to La Madeleine, so that, when the rector of the church, who governs the administration of Salle-aux-Puelles, should die, retire or leave the church, the prior of La Madeleine should take corporal possession of it and Salle-aux-Puelles in perpetuity. Gregory instructs the bishop of Paris to ensure that [in future] there are as many chaplains and ministers in the church of Saint-Julien as there are now and is the custom, that divine offices are fulfilled in the church, and that the sick in the house are received and nourished as previously.

[ADSM, H-Dépôt 1, A39 (original; *vidimus* within copy of letters of Aymeri, bishop of Paris; ?eighteenth-century copy)]

30. Henry II, king of England (1154–89), duke of Normandy (1150–89)

(a) n.d. (1156–April 1166/ ?1156–May 1165; original *vidimus* of Pierre du Busc, keeper of the seal of obligations of the *vicomté* of Rouen, 30 August 1424, also containing the charter of John de Préaux), at Rouen

Henry II confirms the agreement made between the lepers of Mont-aux-Malades and Osbert, lord of Préaux. Annually on the feast of St Michael, Osbert and his heirs must deliver to the lepers 60 measures of barley from the mill of Longpaon, in return for the lepers' peaceful acceptance of Osbert's claim of half the mill, from which they were accustomed to receive 5 measures of wheat and 10 *sous* annually.

[BL, MS Add. charter 11522; edited in *Letters and charters of King Henry II*, no. 2279 (provisional number). See also Langlois, *Histoire*, 88.]

(b) n.d. (February 1165–73/ ?February 1165–March 1170; original *vidimus* of the *vicomte* of Rouen, Thursday after Reminiscere Sunday 1296, and late seventeenth-century [from 1674] abbreviated copy), at Rouen

Henry II donates the church of Saint-Sauveur at Nointot to Mont-aux-Malades, at the request of John de Mara and his wife, patrons of the church. The couple have placed the church in the king's hands at the beseeching of Henry, the king's son. The king also confirms to Mont-aux-Malades the land of Richard de Hayis at Bolleville (Pays de Caux), donated by R. de Thieouville, and the land of Richard de Osqueville at Drosay (*département* of Manche). The first witness of the act is Rotrou of Warwick, archbishop of Rouen.

[ADSM, 25HP3(2) (1296 *vidimus*), 25HP54(2), fo. 1v (late seventeenth-century copy); edited in *Letters and charters of King Henry II*, no. 2280 (provisional number) and Langlois, *Histoire*, 402–3. See also Langlois, *Histoire*, 10.]

(c) n.d. (February 1165–73; original *vidimus* of the *bailli* of Caux, 4 May 1291, and seventeenth-century copy), at Rouen

For the salvation of his grandfather King Henry, his father Geoffrey, count of Anjou, his mother, the Empress Matilda, himself and all his ancestors, Henry II donates a piece of land in the forest of Lillebonne near Bolbec (Pays de Caux) to Mont-aux-Malades.

[ADSM, 25HP3(1) (1291 *vidimus*), 25HP53(1), fo. 1r (seventeenth-century copy); edited in *Letters and charters of King Henry II*, no. 2281 (provisional number)]

(d) n.d. (1170–3/ ?1170–July 1171;[1] original *vidimus* of the *vicomte* of Rouen, Thursday after Reminiscere Sunday 1296, and two seventeenth-century copies), at Quevilly

---

[1] This date range is given in *Letters and charters of King Henry II*. However, Hugh of Amiens, archbishop of Rouen, confirmed Mont-aux-Malades in possession of the church of Beuzeville-la-Grenier in November 1162 (see no. 35 below).

Henry II donates the church of Saint-Martin at Beuzeville-la-Grenier (Pays de Caux) to Mont-aux-Malades, with land in the same parish formerly held by Hugh, his steward, who has returned it to the king so that he may give it to the leper house.

[AN, Paris, S4889B, dossier 13, nos 8 (1296 *vidimus*), 10 (seventeenth-century copy); ADSM, 25HP39 (seventeenth-century copy); edited in *Letters and charters of King Henry II*, no. 2282 (provisional number). See also Langlois, *Histoire*, 11.]

(e) n.d. (May 1172–July 1178/ ?May 1172–May 1175; original, *vidimus* by Simon de Baigneux, *vicomte* of Rouen, 7 Mar. 1386/7, four seventeenth-century copies and one eighteenth-century copy), at Quevilly

For the salvation of his grandfather King Henry, his father Geoffrey, count of Anjou, his mother, the Empress Matilda, himself and all his ancestors, Henry II grants various privileges, rents and lands to the lepers of Mont-aux-Malades. Firstly, the right to hold an annual fair from 1 to 8 September. Both the proceeds from the fair, and the customs on all taxable goods entering Rouen during the fair, will be shared equally between the lepers and himself. Customs on goods at the fair should be charged at the same rate as the customs of Rouen, although the burgesses of Rouen remain exempt from payment of these duties. Secondly, an annual rent of 60 *livres*, 6 *sous*, 8 *deniers roumésins* and 3,000 herrings from the *vicomté* of Rouen and three measures of corn from his mills at Rouen. Thirdly, 140 acres of land in the forest of Lyons, Le Bullin (a hamlet near Mont-aux-Malades) and an area of land in the Pays de Caux between Nointot and the valley road from Bolbec to Mirville (the lordship of La Houssaie-sur-Nointot), 'with all their liberties and free customs' (i.e. the rights of low, middle and high justice).

[ADSM, 25HP1(1)(i) (original); 25HP7(x) (1386/7 *vidimus*) and (xi) (document of 1668 containing two copies); 25HP37 (copy dated 8 June 1768); 25HP54(2), fo. 1r (late seventeenth-century [from 1674] copy); AN, Paris, S4889B, liasse 1, no. 7, fo. 1r–v (1674 copy); edited in *Letters and charters of King Henry II*, no. 2283 (provisional number) and Langlois, *Histoire*, 399–401. See also Langlois, *Histoire*, 7–9, and Six, 'The burgesses of Rouen', 250.]

(f) n.d. (c. 1174–89, in a late seventeenth-century [from 1674] copy, giving the date c. 1176, and another copy made in 1674), at Arques

Henry II pledges to protect the church of Saint-Thomas of Mont-aux-Malades, the lepers, their revenues and possessions, and instructs his men, both ecclesiastical and secular, to do the same. He forbids his men to do any injury to Mont-aux-Malades, or to allow any wrongdoing to be perpetrated against the leper house. He also prohibits pleas regarding property within the leper house's fief, except those brought before himself or his chief justiciar.

[ADSM, 25HP54(2), fo. 1v (late seventeenth-century [from 1674] copy); AN, Paris, S4889B, liasse 1, no. 7, fo. 1v (1674 copy); edited in *Letters and charters of King Henry II*, no. 2284 (provisional number) and Langlois, *Histoire*, 427–8. See also Langlois, *Histoire*, 84.]

(g) n.d. (June 1177–July 1188; copy dated 1396 and seventeenth-century copy), at Guildford

Through love of God and for the salvation of himself and his ancestors, Henry II donates an annual grant of 6,000 herrings from the *prévôté* of Dieppe to the lepers of Mont-aux-Malades.

[ADSM, G851 (Coutumier de Dieppe), fos 64v–65r (1396 copy), G1265 (seventeenth-century copy). Archival information derived from *Letters and charters of King Henry II*, no. 2285 (provisional number). Edited in *Letters and charters of King Henry II*, no. 2285. See also Langlois, *Histoire*, 11.]

(h) n.d. (1180 pipe roll)

Record of a payment of 8 *livres*, 2 *sous* and 8 *deniers* of 'established alms' from the Norman Exchequer to the lepers of Rouen.

[*Pipe rolls of the Exchequer*, 50]

(i) n.d. (April 1185–January 1188), at Cherbourg

For the salvation of his soul and those of his ancestors and successors, Henry II has given to the leprous women of Quevilly, in free and perpetual alms, his enclosure of houses at Quevilly, where he built their lodging. He has also donated 200 *livres* of Anjou per year for the women's sustenance and clothing from the *vicomté* of Rouen (100 *livres* on the feast of St Michael and 100 *livres* at Easter), until he assigns them money from lands or rents of churches elsewhere. He has given them the meadow of Quevilly which Marinus de Hosa asserted, the right to put their beasts to pasture in the forest [of Rouvray], exemption from paying pannage for their pigs in the forest, and the right to take there the wood that they need for heating and repairing their houses. He also grants them exemption from land and water taxes for [transporting] their wine and other necessary things, and various other exemptions to them and their men.

[ADSM, 27HP95 ?(fourteenth-century copy made under the seal of the *mairie* of Rouen); BM, Rouen, Chartrier de la ville, Tiroir 109, dossier 1, doc. (ii), fos 4r–5r (?sixteenth-century copy); ADSM, H-Dépôt 1, A39 (?seventeenth-century printed copy); edited in *Letters and charters of King Henry II*, no. 2112 (provisional number); *Recueil des actes*, ii. 296–7 (no. 678); Farin, *Histoire*, ii/5, 121–2 (translated into French); Duchemin, *Petit-Quevilly*, 229 (after Farin)]

31. Henry, the Young King (1170–83)

n.d. (c. 1173–early 1183, original; *vidimus* of the *vicomte* of Rouen, Thursday after Reminiscere Sunday 1296; seventeenth-century copy of the *vidimus*), at Quevilly

The Young King Henry gives notice that, at his request, John de Mara has given the church of Nointot to Mont-aux-Malades in perpetual alms.

[ADSM, 25HP7(ix) (original); 25HP3(2)(i) (1296 *vidimus*), (ii) (seventeenth-century copy of the *vidimus*); edited in *Recueil des actes*, introduction, 257; Langlois, *Histoire*, 404. See also Langlois, *Histoire*, 11, and Smith, 'Henry II's heir', 324 (no. 29).]

32. Henry, prior of La Madeleine hospital, Rouen, and the whole community

Monday after the feast of St Remigius, October 1261 (original and seventeenth-century copy)

The prior and community of Mont-aux-Malades have done special grace to the community at La Madeleine with regard to their leprous brother, Canon Roger, and leprous sister, Haisia, who were received into Mont-aux-Malades on the Sunday after the feast of St Remigius, 1261 [i.e. the day before this charter was issued]. At the request of Prior Henry of La Madeleine, the prior and community of Mont-aux-Malades have granted that Brother Roger is to have the same entitlement to food and drink as a brother of Mont-aux-Malades, and sister Haisia is to have the same entitlement as a sister of Mont-aux-Malades. The community at La Madeleine grants to Mont-aux-Malades repayment of the goods which the two individuals take at the leper house (as long as they live), if the community at Mont-aux-Malades wishes to receive this reimbursement.

[AN, Paris, S4889B, dossier 13, nos 17 (seventeenth-century copy), 18 (original). See also Langlois, *Histoire*, 123.]

33. Henry de Sully, fifth abbot of Fécamp (1139–88)

1154 (original and seventeenth-century copy), at Fécamp

At the request of Henry II, Hugh of Amiens, archbishop of Rouen, the Empress Matilda and the burgesses of Rouen, with the consent of the whole chapter of Fécamp, Henry de Sully has granted 4 acres of land in the fief of the priory of Saint-Gervais, Rouen, to the lepers of Rouen (Mont-aux-Malades). Two acres are Henry's own gift and 2 acres are the gift of Roger, his predecessor as abbot of Fécamp. In return for conceding the grant, the prior of Saint-Gervais is to receive 2 pounds of pepper, 2 tapers worth 11 *sous* each and 1 pound of incense annually. The grant is confirmed by Roger, priest of Saint-Gervais.

[AN, Paris, S4889B, liasse 1, nos 4 (original), 5 (seventeenth-century copy). See also Langlois, *Histoire*, 12. The priory of Saint-Gervais was a dependency of the abbey of Fécamp.]

34. Honorius III, pope (1216–27)

10 June 1219 (original), at Rome

Honorius gives greetings to his beloved daughters in Christ, the prioress and religious women of the leper house of Quevilly. He agrees to their petitions, forbidding anyone from demanding tithes from them for their gardens and orchards.

[ADSM, H-Dépôt 1, A39]

35. Hugh of Amiens, archbishop of Rouen (1130–64)

26 October 1162 (in an original *vidimus* of the *vicomte* of Rouen, date lost [late thirteenth century], and in an original *vidimus* of the official of Rouen, 1301)

Archbishop Hugh confirms the clerics of Mont-aux-Malades and their successors in their possession of the church of Saint-Pierre de Carville, the chapel of Saint-Ouen de Longpaon and the church of Saint-Martin de Beuzeville-la-Grenier.

[ADSM, 25HP36(ii) (late thirteenth-century *vidimus*), (vi) (1301 *vidimus*)]

36. Hugh de Martainville

November 1217 (in an original *vidimus* of the *vicomte* of Rouen, 1293)

Hugh has given to Mont-aux-Malades, in pure and perpetual alms, 15 *sous*, 1 capon of annual rent due from a tenement near the church of Saint-Hilaire, Rouen.

[ADSM, 25HP1(8)(xviii). See also Langlois, *Histoire*, 93–4.]

37. Hugh du Monastère, citizen of Rouen, of the parish of Saint-Martin-sur-Renelle, Rouen

May 1262 (Hugh's original act), April 1262 (original act of the official of Rouen)

Inspired by charity and for the salvation of his soul and those of his ancestors, Hugh has donated to Mont-aux-Malades 20 *sous* annual rent (7 *sous*, plus 13 *sous* which Mont-aux-Malades previously held from Hugh's tenement in the parish of Saint-Martin-sur-Renelle).

[ADSM, 25HP1(8)(xxi), (xxii)]

38. Hugh de Sahurs, rector of the church of Saint-Jacques of Moulineaux

n.d. (original, 1236–44, probably September 1240)

Hugh has sworn obedience and reverence to P., archbishop of Rouen [Peter de Colle-mezzo]. He confirms that he will serve in the church of Saint-Jacques of Moulineaux, and will observe its rights. He will not alienate the church's property, and he will recover any property that has been alienated. He states that he has not made any gifts in order to be presented to the church.

[ADSM, H-Dépôt 1, F1]

39. James Le Breton, lieutenant general of Mr de Chateillon, inquisitor of waters, islands, forests, warrens, rivers and appurtenances in the kingdom of France

17 January 1385 (in French, ?seventeenth-century printed copy), at Rouen

James Le Breton gives greetings to the verderer of the forest of Rouvray, or his lieutenant. In Rouen and the *vicomté* of Rouen, certain parties have been prevented from enjoying their rights to royal waters, forests, warrens and appurtenances, until they can produce the charters or letters by which they have enjoyed them in the past. The prior, brothers and sisters of the Hôtel-Dieu of Rouen [La Madeleine hospital] have shown him letters stating the rights which the sick women of Quevilly were accustomed to enjoy in the forest of Rouvray, by reason of their house called Salle-aux-Puelles. King Charles [v] gave Salle-aux-Puelles with these rights to the Hôtel-Dieu, as can be seen by the *vidimus* of his letters, and by the resignation made by the attorney of Walter Le Sage, priest, master and governor of Salle-aux-Puelles. James Le Breton orders the verderer to allow the prior, brothers and sisters of the Hôtel-Dieu to enjoy the rights belonging to Salle-aux-Puelles, in the manner contained in the letters of King Charles, provided that they do not abuse or exceed these.

[ADSM, H-Dépôt 1, A39. See also Duchemin, *Petit-Quevilly*, 232–3: Walter Le Sage, secular priest, held the benefice of the church of Saint-Julien and was master of Salle-aux-Puelles in 1366. After Charles v's donation of Salle-aux-Puelles to La Madeleine that year, he initially retained his appointment, but resigned it in an act of 4 Aug. 1384.]

40. James Le Petit and his wife Alina

1226 (original act of James Le Petit and original confirmation by Theobald of Amiens, archbishop of Rouen [1222–9])

James and Alina have granted 20 *sous* of annual rent to Mont-aux-Malades due from the tenement which Bertin, grandson of Bartholomew Le Cras, canon of Rouen (1207–23), holds from them. The tenement is situated in the parish of Saint-Maclou, between the Aubette river, the tenement of Ralph, cleric, and the land of Matilda Le Gros (the wife of Matthew Le Gros, mayor of Rouen in 1195, 1198–1200). The prior and brothers of Mont-aux-Malades have given James and Alina 10 *livres* of Tours in recognition of this grant.

[ADSM, 25HP6]

41. John de Beuzevillette, prior of Mont-aux-Malades (1252–88)

(a) May 1259 (in a late seventeenth-century [from 1674] copy)

With 'the whole community ... both the canons and the sick', John renews Prior Nicholas's act establishing a fraternity arrangement between Mont-aux-Malades and the palmers of Rouen.

[ADSM, 25HP 54(2), fos 1v–2r. Two of the palmers, their master, William Compivo and their *échevin* Robert Le Tondeur, witness John's act; Langlois, *Histoire*, 3–4.]

(b) February 1280 (original)

John and the community of Mont-aux-Malades have granted a homestead of land in the parish of Saint-Laurent, Rouen, to Geoffrey Belleville and his brother Robert, for 25 *sous* of Tours annual rent.

[ADSM, 25HP1(17)(vii)]

42. John, king of England (1199–1216)

16 October 1200, at Clarendon

John takes the church of Mont-aux-Malades and the lepers there into his protection, and orders his archbishops to do the same. He forbids any pleas regarding Mont-aux-Malades's tenements, except in the presence of himself or his chief justiciar, as is stated in the letters patent of King Henry, his predecessor.

[Edited in *Rotuli chartarum in turri Londinensi*, i/1, p. 76. See also Langlois, *Histoire*, 89–90.]

43. John Hardi, of the parish of Saint-Martin-du-Pont, Rouen

Monday after the circumcision of the Lord, 1304 (in a *vidimus* of the official of Rouen, 1304, stating that John is now deceased, in an original *vidimus* of the official of Rouen, 1353, and in another *vidimus* of the official of Rouen, 1304, Friday after the commission of St Paul the Apostle)

John's testament, naming numerous religious and secular communities, individuals and institutions as beneficiaries. These include: the church of Saint-Martin-du-Pont, Rouen; Rouen cathedral; the poor at La Madeleine hospital; the hospital of the rue Saint-Ouen; the hospital of the rue Saint-Martin-du-Pont; the Brothers Minor of Rouen, in whose church he chooses to be buried; the priory of Mont-aux-Malades (20 *sous*); the priory of Salle-aux-Puelles (10 *sous*); the lepers of the four gates of Rouen (20 *sous*); the lepers of Répainville (5 *sous*); the lepers of Darnétal (5 *sous*); 'the poor lepers who flock together at Rouen on Good Friday' (20 *sous* of Tours); the poor pilgrims 'on the day after Easter Day' (20 *sous*); 'the poor lepers who flock together at Rouen on the Monday, Tuesday, Wednesday and Thursday of the Ascension' (20 *sous* of Tours); the poor prisoners in the castle of Rouen (20 *sous* of Tours); the poor prisoners in the *curia* of the official of Rouen (10 *sous*); the poor prisoners in the mayor's prison (10 *sous*); the poor 'sitting' in Rouen cathedral; the confraternity of the cathedral (10 *sous*); the confraternity of the church of Saint-Martin-du-Pont (10 *sous*). John also specifies an alms distribution at the cathedral on behalf of lepers (5 *sous*), and, for the salvation of himself and his wife Joanna, donates a furnished bed for the use of the poor at La Madeleine hospital. Finally, he donates 20 *livres* of Tours annual rent to establish a chapel and priest at the church of Saint-Martin-du-Pont, for the salvation of his soul and those of his friends and successors.

[ADSM, G1236, G7137; partially transcribed in Tabuteau, 'Léproseries', 205. The *Livre des Jurés* of the abbey of Saint-Ouen lists the tenure of land at Quincampoix, north-east of Rouen, by John Hardi between 1299 and 1302; this man could be synonymous with the John Hardi whose testament was drawn up in 1304. See *Un Censier normand du XIIIe siècle: le Livre des Jurés de l'abbaye Saint-Ouen de Rouen*, ed. Denise Angers, Catherine Bébéar and Henri Dubois, Paris 2001, pp. vii–viii, 369.]

44. John de Hodenc

n.d. (*c.* 1174–1200; original)

John's gift of land and rent at Saint-Gervais, Rouen to three religious houses in perpetual alms: Mont-aux-Malades, La Madeleine hospital and the abbey of Sainte-Marie at Beaubec. He makes the gift with the consent of his wife Alix (de Préaux) and their son Giles, for the salvation of their souls and the souls of their children, ancestors and friends. The land returns 13 *livres* annually: on the feast of Saint Remigius 4 *livres* are to be paid to Mont-aux-Malades, 4 *livres* to La Madeleine hospital, and 100 *sous* to the monks of Beaubec. The three religious houses are to come into possession of these gifts upon the death of John or his wife, who holds this land through marriage.

[ADSM, 25HP1(24)(i). See also Arnoux, 'Les Origines', 146.]

45. John Le Moutardier and his wife Alicia, of the parish of Saint-Maclou, Rouen

September 1271 (original act of the official of Rouen)

John and Alicia have taken in fief and perpetual hereditary possession from Mont-aux-Malades, for 74 *sous* annual rent, a tenement in Saint-Maclou parish, situated between the land of Godard Quenousart and that of Alicia de Boes.

[ADSM, 25HP6]

46. John Le Vilein, brother of the late Roger Le Vilein, citizen of Rouen

1323, Saturday after the feast of St Clement (original act of the *bailli* of Rouen, in French)

In order for his brother Laurence Le Vilein to be received as a brother at Mont-aux-Malades, and to enjoy the goods of the house like one of the other brothers of his condition, John has donated to Mont-aux-Malades 4 *livres* of rent in perpetuity, and 16 *livres* of rent during Laurence's life.

[ADSM, 25HP1. See also Tabuteau, 'Léproseries', 128.]

47. John du Mont-Guérout of the parish of Beuzevillette (near Bolbec, Pays de Caux)

February 1278 (original)

For 30 *sous* John has sold to Mont-aux-Malades 3 *sous* of rent which William Sochon paid him annually from his (William's) tenement in the parish of Beuzevillette, and all rights he (John) held to the property. William and his heirs will now pay the rent to Mont-aux-Malades without any opposition from John or his heirs.

[ADSM, 25HP1(1)(vi)]

48. John d'Offranville

n.d. (1191–1218, probably c. 1210–18, in an original *vidimus* of the *vicomte* of Rouen, 1293)

John and his heirs are held to deliver 32 *sous* (current money) annual rent to Mont-aux-Malades from the tenement which Robert de Saint-Jacques gave to Mont-aux-Malades.

[ADSM, 25HP1(8)(xviii)]

49. John du Parc

1316 (original act of the *bailli* of Rouen, in French)

For the cause of his brother Peter du Parc being received as a brother there, John has donated 30 *sous* of rent in perpetuity to Mont-aux-Malades.

[ADSM, 25HP1. See also Tabuteau, 'Léproseries', 128.]

50. John de Préaux

n.d. (from c. 1174: late twelfth or early thirteenth century; original *vidimus* of Pierre du Busc, keeper of the seal of obligations of the *vicomté* of Rouen, 30 Aug. 1424), at Beaulieu

For the salvation of his soul and those of his father, mother and ancestors, John has donated to Mont-aux-Malades 60 measures of barley annually from the mills of Crevon and Launay, which the leper house previously received from the mill of Longpaon.

[BL, MS Add. Charter 11522. See also Langlois, *Histoire*, 88. John, the son of Alix, daughter of Osbert de Préaux (see Arnoux, 'Les Origines', 146), reconfirms his grandfather's gift, for which see no. 30(a).]

51. Laurence Bouguenel

April 1233 (original)

Laurence has granted in perpetuity to the prior and brothers of Mont-aux-Malades the 9 *sous* annual rent which his mother Laurentia Bouguenel gave them when she entered their house.

[ADSM, 25HP1(17)(viii)]

52. Laurence Chamberlain, knight, Louis IX's *panetier royal* at Rouen, lord of Saint-Aignan

(a) May 1278 (original)

Laurence has granted 5 *sous* of Tours, 5 capons of annual rent to Mont-aux-Malades, due from a tenement in the parish of Saint-Jacques of Mont-aux-Malades, in the leper house's fief. For 15 *sous* of Tours annual rent due at Barengerville, he has also exchanged with Mont-aux-Malades half an acre of land between Le Tronquai and the *villa* of Mont-aux-Malades.

[ADSM, 25HP10(xxv). See also Langlois, *Histoire*, 97.]

(b) August 1289 (original)

With the consent of his wife Matilda, Laurence has given in perpetual farm to Mont-aux-Malades his entire fief which he held from the king of France at Saint-Aignan (and Le Tronquai). Mont-aux-Malades is to hold the fief from the king of France as Laurence did, for 23 *livres* of Tours annual rent, 'with the buildings on the farm … at Saint-Aignan and elsewhere in the said parish'. In exchange, Mont-aux-Malades has granted to Laurence and his heirs 10 *livres* of Tours annual rent, and its inheritance at Sotteville, near Pont-de-l'Arche and Igouville, and at Les Authieux. This grant excludes some fields at Sotteville which Laurence and Matilda already hold; Laurence and his heirs are held to pay 3 *sous* of Tours annual rent to the abbey of Saint-Ouen, Rouen, for this land at Sotteville. The community of Mont-aux-Malades has also granted the revenues and men which it held at Pîtres to Laurence.

[ADSM, 25HP1(4)(iii). See also Farin, *Histoire*, ii/6, pp. 26, 29, and Langlois, *Histoire*, 97, describing the fief at Saint-Aignan as the farm of Étouteville.]

53. Leiarda, daughter of Gondoin

Date lost (1223: witnessed by Peter de Quevilly as mayor of Rouen [1222–3]; later hand on verso gives the date 1223; original)

Leiarda owes Mont-aux-Malades 5 *sous* of rent (usual money at Rouen) from a tenement in the rue Brasière, Rouen, situated next to the land of Alix de Cailli, Peter Luce and John Blondel.

[ADSM, 25HP1(10)(iii)]

54. Louis IX, king of France (1226–70)

March 1269, at Villeneuve-le-Roi, near Sens (in an original *vidimus* of Philip III, May 1274, at Gisors, and in an original *vidimus* of the official of Rouen, 1277, witnessing Philip III's *vidimus*)

Louis IX confirms Mont-aux-Malades' possessions.

[ADSM, 25HP7(vii) (*vidimus* of Philip III); 25HP11(1)(iv) (?seventeenth-century copy of Philip III's *vidimus*); 25HP46 (1732 copy of Philip III's *vidimus*); AN, Paris, S4889B, dossier 13, nos 15 (seventeenth-century copy of 1277 *vidimus*), 16 (1277 *vidimus*); edited in *Cartulaire normand*, 342 (no. 1226). See also Langlois, *Histoire*, 95.]

55. Louis, son of William, son of Gondoin

n.d. (1195 or 1198–1200; original)

For 45 ½ *livres* of Anjou, with the consent of his grandsons Robert and William de Jafres, Louis has sold to Prior Robert of Mont-aux-Malades, and the brothers healthy and sick serving God there, 61 *sous* of rent due from various fiefs at Rouen, with whatever rights he held regarding these fiefs.

[ADSM, 25HP1(8)(xv)]

56. Martin de Quevilly, citizen of Rouen

1291 (the Sunday following the feast of SS Bartholomew and Ouen) (original charter in French of the *vicomte* of Rouen, giving notice of Martin's gift)

For God, his salvation and that of his ancestors, Martin has donated to Mont-aux-Malades six verges of meadow which he held in the parish of Saint-Martin at Canteleu, between the meadow of William de Croisset and that of the priory of Saint-Lô, Rouen.

[ADSM, 25HP47(7)(xiv)]

57. Matilda Le Changeur, widow of Renaud Le Changeur

1228 (original charter of Theobald of Amiens, archbishop of Rouen, giving notice of Matilda's gift)

With the consent of her son Michael, for the salvation of her soul, Matilda has given in perpetuity to Mont-aux-Malades 22 *sous* annual rent due from a tenement in the Malpalu area of Rouen, 'to make the light of the altar of the Holy Trinity in the church of St Thomas the Martyr' [therefore, to supply candles to illuminate this altar in Mont-aux-Malades' church].

[ADSM, 25HP6]

58. Matilda Piguet, widow, of the parish of Saint-Gervais, Rouen

Thursday after Easter, 1296 (original act in French of the *vicomte* of Rouen)

Matilda has donated to Mont-aux-Malades, 'for the sake of God, in alms, in order to find her living there sufficiently for as long as she should live', two pieces of land at Saint-Gervais, 22 *sous* annual rent, and a piece of land in the parish of Saint-Aignan, situated between the land of Mont-aux-Malades and that of Richard des Hayes.

[ADSM, 25HP1(24)(vii)]

59. Matthew de Neuville

n.d. (*c.* 1174–1200; original)

In perpetual alms, for the salvation of his soul, Matthew has given to Mont-aux-Malades a measure of salt ... and 6 *sous* of rent due at Montivilliers, 'towards the lighting of the church of St Thomas the Martyr'.

[ADSM, 25HP1(20)]

60. Nicholas de la Commune, cleric

1262 (original *vidimus* of the official of Rouen, witnessing the deceased Nicholas's testament, bearing the seals of the prior of Mont-aux-Malades [John de Beuzevillette, prior 1254–88], Roger, priest of Écauville and Richard du Vicomté, who are Nicholas's executors)

Nicholas bequeaths to God and Mont-aux-Malades, for his salvation and that of his ancestors, 50 *sous* of annual rent (mostly due from the parish of Saint-Nicolas-de-Bellevue) at his death, for the pittance of the sick and other members of the community at Mont-aux-Malades. He also donates a silver cup, and chooses to be buried at Mont-aux-Malades.

[ADSM, 25HP3]

61. Nicholas, prior of Mont-aux-Malades (c. 1135–73)

n.d. (c. 1135–73, probably c. 1145–50; in a renewal by John de Beuzevillette, prior of Mont-aux-Malades, May 1259, recorded in a late seventeenth-century [from 1674] copy; also another seventeenth-century copy, in which Geoffrey of Anjou gives notice of Nicholas's act)

Nicholas and the whole community of Mont-aux-Malades have taken the brothers and sisters of the fraternity of the palmers of Rouen into their brotherhood, for the performance of masses, vigils and orations in the leper house church. This is agreed on condition that the palmers process annually to Mont-aux-Malades on the day of the Finding of the Holy Cross (3 May), with an alms contribution from their profits through pilgrimage and work, and 7 pints of wine. When one of the palmers dies, the prior and community of Mont-aux-Malades pledge to celebrate full service for the individual as if for one of their own deceased. This act was drawn up 'in the chapter of the sick', in the presence of the prior, the canons and the sick.

[ADSM, 25HP54(2), fos 1v–2r (late seventeenth-century [from 1674] copy); 25HP46 (second seventeenth-century copy). See also Langlois, *Histoire*, 3–4.]

62. Nicholas Pigache, citizen of Rouen, mayor of Rouen in 1208–9, 1219–20

July 1219, at Déville (notification by Robert Poulain, archbishop of Rouen [1208–21], in an original *vidimus* of the official of Rouen, 1249)

Nicholas has donated 10 *livres* of Tours annual rent to sustain a priest to celebrate mass daily at the altar of St Mary Magdalene in the church at Mont-aux-Malades, in the presence of female lepers, for the salvation of Nicholas, his wife, father, mother and other ancestors. He has also given a rent of 40 *sous* of Tours to have a lamp burning constantly before this altar. The prior and community of Mont-aux-Malades have agreed that the priest established by Nicholas should have the same entitlement to food and drink as the leper house's canons.

[ADSM, 25HP10(viii). This gift resulted in the establishment of a chantry chapel for the Pigache family in the church of Saint-Thomas at Mont-aux-

Malades: *Regestrum*, 513; *Register*, 585. According to Langlois (*Histoire*, 99–100), in 1285 (on the Saturday before the feast of St Mary Magdalene), Nicholas's son, John Pigache (mayor of Rouen in 1255–6, 1262–3, 1271–2, 1272–3) increased the family chaplain's stipend by 30 *sous* per year. In 1301 Martin Pigache, Nicholas's grandson, granted the canons of Mont-aux-Malades the right to appoint the chaplain from amongst themselves.]

63. Nicholas de Puteo

1205 (original)

On the occasion of his son Nicholas taking the habit at Mont-aux-Malades, Nicholas has donated to the leper house 10 *sous* of annual rent in free, pure, perpetual alms, for love of God and the salvation of himself and his ancestors. The rent is due from two houses held by Nicholas de Busco and his son-in-law Ralph, in front of Nicholas de Puteo's house in the parish of Saint-Pierre-le-Portier, Rouen.

[ADSM, 25HP6]

64. The official of Rouen (unnamed)

1260 (original)

The official resolves a dispute between G., prior of Salle-aux-Puelles, and Durand Rebors, who had claimed the patronage of the church of Saint-Jacques of Moulineaux. Durand has acknowledged that G.'s predecessor as prior was presented to this church by the archbishop of Rouen or his vicar. This presentation was ceded legally, and Durand now wishes for the prior to have possession of the church.

[ADSM, H-Dépôt 1, F1]

65. The official of Rouen (unnamed)

1399 (original)

The official gives notice of a dispute between the prior and brothers of La Madeleine, Rouen, and Matthew Machon, priest, rector of the parish church of Moulineaux, regarding the necessary repairs to the chancel of the church. He establishes that La Madeleine is to pay for two thirds of the repairs, and the rector for one third.

[ADSM, H-Dépôt 1, F1. La Madeleine came into possession of the church of Moulineaux when Salle-aux-Puelles was unified with it in 1366.]

66. Osbert Puchart, citizen of Rouen

1201 (in an original *vidimus* of the *vicomte* of Rouen, 1293)

Osbert has taken in fief and hereditary possession from Mont-aux-Malades a house in the parish of Saint-Herbland, Rouen, in return for 6 *livres* annual rent from himself and his heirs.

[ADSM, 25HP1(4)(ii)]

67. Peter de Collemezzo, archbishop of Rouen (1236–44)

(a) 1240 (original), at Rouen

Archbishop Peter gives greetings to the dean of Rouen. Since he has bestowed the church of Saint-Jacques of Moulineaux on Hugh de Sahurs, at the request of the prior and community of Salle-aux-Puelles, he instructs the dean to appoint Hugh to the church and put him in possession of it. He also orders the dean, with two priests from the deanery, to make an inventory of the church's revenues, books, vestments and other ornaments.

[ADSM, H-Dépôt 1, F1]

(b) September 1240 (original), at Déville

Archbishop Peter gives notice that there have been many complaints to himself and his predecessors about the churches of Sahurs and Grand-Couronne, and the chapel of Saint-Jacques of Moulineaux, regarding the flooding of the fields. ... On the advice of the chapter of Rouen, in the presence of the prior of Salle-aux-Puelles, the priest of [Grand-]Couronne, and the rector of Sahurs, he has ordered that Saint-Jacques of Moulineaux is to become a parish church, and the parishioners of Grand-Couronne and Sahurs living at Moulineaux should be its parishioners. Because the church of Sahurs is much disadvantaged by this measure, he orders that the priest of Moulineaux should pay the priest of Sahurs 20 *sous* of Tours annually.

[The chapel at Moulineaux was made into a parish church because the residents of Moulineaux were unable to access the churches of Sahurs and Grand-Couronne at times of flooding.]

[ADSM, H-Dépôt 1, F1]

68. [Peter Saimel], *bailli* of Rouen (1298–1302)

(a) 1299, during the Easter Exchequer (original)

The *bailli* gives greetings to G. [William de Flavacourt], archbishop of Rouen. There has been a dispute regarding the patronage of the church of Saint-Jacques of Moulineaux, between the king of France [Philip IV] and Walter, prior of Salle-aux-Puelles and the sisters there. The *bailli* gives notice that the prior and sisters and their attorney have been judged to hold the patronage of the church, and should be brought into corporal possession of it.

[ADSM, H-Dépôt 1, F1]

(b) 1299, during the Easter Exchequer, at Rouen (original)

The *bailli* has heard the supplication of the prior and the procurator of Salle-aux-Puelles, regarding the fact that the king has prevented them from enjoying their right of patronage and presentation with regard to the church of Saint-Jacques of Moulineaux. He establishes that the right of patronage and presentation to this church does belong to Salle-aux-Puelles.

[ADSM, H-Dépôt 1, F1. On Peter Saimel, *bailli* of Rouen, see Maurice Veyrat, *Essai chronologique et biographique sur les baillis de Rouen (de 1171 à 1790)*, Rouen 1953, 53–4, 261.]

69. Peter de Saint-Gille

1312, Monday before Palm Sunday (original, in French)

By necessity of his disease, Peter has made the following contract with Mont-aux-Malades. In return for being received in the community of the sick, to be with them for the rest of his life, and to enjoy the goods of the house as one of the sick brothers, he has given to Mont-aux-Malades 10 *livres* of Tours and two adjacent houses in the parish of Saint-Martin-sur-Renelle, Rouen. However, the sick from his parish [presumably Saint-Martin-sur-Renelle] cannot claim a privilege [to enter Mont-aux-Malades] because he has been received in the community of the sick.

[ADSM, 25HP1. See also Tabuteau, 'Léproseries', 118.]

70. Peter de Saint-Jacques and his wife Avicia

July 1226 (original act of Theobald of Amiens, archbishop of Rouen)

Archbishop Theobald gives notice that, in his *curia* in the presence of Alan Brito, official of Rouen, Peter de Saint-Jacques and his wife Avicia have donated 5 *sous* annual rent due from the parish of Saint-Patrice, Rouen to Mont-aux-Malades in perpetual alms, for the sake of their souls and those of their benefactors and friends. William, prior, and Restondus and Andrew, canons of Mont-aux-Malades have agreed that they and their successors will retain ½ *livre* of this rent to make a candle to burn night and day once a year in perpetuity, in honour of St Martha the Martyr, sister of St Mary Magdalene, on Martha's saint's day (fourth calends of August). Inspired by charity, the said prior and canons of Mont-aux-Malades have given Peter and Avicia 40 *sous* of Tours.

[ADSM, 25HP1(26)(viii)]

71. Petronilla de Carville, of the parish of Saint-Martin-du-Pont, Rouen

January 1254 (original act of the official of Rouen)

For 30 *sous* of Tours, with the consent of her husband, William Anglici, Petronilla has sold to Mont-aux-Malades 4 ½ *sous* (usual money) annual rent due from a meadow in the parish of Saint-Hilaire, Rouen, situated between the Robec river and the land of Ralph Relant, stretching from the meadow of the abbey of Saint-Amand to the land of Herbert.

[ADSM, 25HP6]

72. Petronilla, daughter of Ralph de Malo Alneto, carpenter, of the parish of Saint-Michel in the *Vieux Marché*, Rouen

August 1256 (original act of the official of Rouen)

For the salvation of her soul and those of her ancestors, Petronilla has donated to Mont-aux-Malades, in perpetual alms, her tenement in the parish of Saint-Patrice, Rouen, situated between the land of Ralph Gorge and that of Roman Le Fondeur, with 24 *sous* (usual money) annual rent from the tenement of Roman Le Fondeur, and 8 *sous*, 6 *deniers* (usual money) annual rent from the tenement of William Le Blond, situated in the rue Stoupato, Rouen.

[ADSM, 25HP1(26)(xxvii)]

73. Philip Augustus, king of France (1180–1223)

(a) November 1207 (in an original *vidimus* of the *bailli* of Caux, 4 May 1291, witnessing a *vidimus* of the *vicomte* of Rouen, 1290, witnessing Philip Augustus' act), at Montargis

Inspired by holy piety, Philip Augustus has taken Mont-aux-Malades, with all things pertaining to it, under his protection. He has ordered all his *baillis* to maintain and defend Mont-aux-Malades and all its possessions, and not to trouble the leper house unduly. He also wishes that Mont-aux-Malades should peacefully hold all things which it held during the reigns of Henry II and Richard I, kings of England, without being troubled.

[Léopold Delisle, *Catalogue des actes de Philippe-Auguste*, Paris 1856, 246 (no. 1062); *Recueil des actes de Philippe Auguste, roi de France*, ed. H.-François Delaborde and others, Paris 1916–2005, iii. 67–8 (no. 1006). See also Langlois, *Histoire*, 90 (where Philip Augustus' act is erroneously dated to 7 November 1200).]

(b) *c.* 1210

Philip Augustus confirms grants of alms at Rouen: 8 *livres*, 2 *sous*, 8 *deniers* to Mont-aux-Malades, 40 *livres* to La Madeleine hospital, and 2 *sous* to the leprous women of Salle-aux-Puelles.

[Edited in *Cartulaire normand*, 33 (no. 210)]

74. Philip III, king of France (1270–85)

(a) 1278 (in an act of William de Flavacourt, archbishop of Rouen)

For an annual rent of 180 *livres*, Philip III has granted to Mont-aux-Malades in perpetuity the barony of Fréville (in the Pays de Caux, midway between Mont-aux-Malades and Nointot). These estates consist of 218 acres of cultivable land, 38 acres of fields and 40 acres of woods. The annual feudal dues previously delivered to the king are now made over to Mont-aux-Malades: 30 *livres*, 1 barrel of barley, 76 barrels and 2 bushels of oats, 4 barrels of wheat, 2,720 eggs, 5 barrels of salt, 24 hens, 387 turkeys, and 2 strong beech trees from the felling of trees in the forêt du Trait (next to the barony of Fréville). In addition, the abbey of Saint-Wandrille will deliver to Mont-aux-Malades (annually, by virtue of an interest the abbey holds in the lordship of Fréville) 12 white loaves, 1 *setier* (approximately 8 pints) of wine, 1 *setier* of beer and a quantity of beef and lamb. Philip has granted the right of low justice at Fréville to Mont-aux-Malades, but retains that of high justice, and the patronage of the church, for himself.

[Description derived from Langlois, *Histoire*, 95–6.]

(b) Aug. 1281, at Paris (original and eighteenth-century copy)

Inspired by piety and through love of God, for the cure of his soul and the souls of Queen Isabelle, formerly his wife, King Louis his father and his other ancestors, Philip III has granted to Mont-aux-Malades in perpetuity the patronage of the church of Saint-Martin at Fréville. On the first vacancy of the church and thenceforth, two canons of Mont-aux-Malades should be installed there, one as parish priest and the other to celebrate mass daily for the king: a mass of the holy spirit while he is alive, and a mass of the dead after his death. In addition (after the king's death), the prior and brothers of Mont-aux-Malades must commemorate Philip's anniversary annually in their monastery.

[ASDM, 25HP7(ii) (original), 25HP1(9)(v) (copy dated October 1714). See also Langlois, *Histoire*, 96–7.]

75. Philip IV, king of France (1285–1314)

(a) September 1290, at Paris (an original *vidimus* witnessing the act [in French] of the *bailli* of Rouen, April 1290 [during the Easter Exchequer]), at Rouen

At the command of the Exchequer of Saint-Michel in 1289, for the profit of the king, the *bailli* of Rouen has granted the farm of Saint-Victor at Saint-Aignan in perpetual farm to Mont-aux-Malades, in return for an annual rent of 4 *livres*, 8 *sous* of Tours to be delivered to the king. Mont-aux-Malades is entitled to claim various rents from individuals who hold land and property on the farm. The king retains the right of high justice. Philip IV confirms that he wishes these things.

[ADSM, 25HP1(7). See also Farin, *Histoire*, ii/6, 29.]

(b) December 1296, at the castle of Lyons (original)

Inspired by piety, for the salvation of his soul and that of his beloved wife Jeanne, Philip IV donates the patronage of the church of Saint-Aignan, near Rouen, to Mont-aux-Malades in perpetuity, with all its profits and revenues. One of the canons of Mont-aux-Malades is to serve in the church as parish priest. The religious of Mont-aux-Malades are held to celebrate (in the church of Saint-Aignan) a daily mass of the holy spirit on behalf of Philip and his wife while they live, and a daily requiem for the sake of their souls after their deaths. Following their deaths, the religious of Mont-aux-Malades must also celebrate Philip and Jeanne's anniversaries in the leper house church.

[ADSM, 25HP7(i); edited in Langlois, *Histoire*, 431–2. See also Langlois, *Histoire*, 98, and Farin, *Histoire*, ii/6, 29.]

(c) 1300 (the Wednesday before Palm Sunday), at Paris (original)

Philip IV gives greetings to the *bailli* of Caux. He has received a complaint from the prior and brothers of Mont-aux-Malades, regarding the full powers of justice that they have been accustomed to hold, through the alms of Henry II, king of England, at Nointot and other towns and territories in the surrounding area. They have held these rights for a long time, according to Henry II's charter. However, the *bailli* of Caux is hindering them in the enjoyment of their rights, and they are greatly troubled by this. Philip orders the *bailli* to inspect their charter: if he finds that their claims are correct, he must cease from this hindrance and harrassment, and permit the prior and brothers to enjoy their rights of justice. He must also refrain from making such unjustified claims in the future.

[ADSM, 25HP7(iii). See also Langlois, *Histoire*, 102–3.]

76. Philip VI, king of France (1328–50)

(a) 15 February 1330 (original copy in French made under the seal of obligations of the *vicomté* of Rouen), at Saint-Germain-en-Laye

Philip VI gives greetings to John Le Veneur, master of his forests, and the *bailli* of Gisors. The prior and the four communities of Mont-aux-Malades, both healthy and leprous, have appealed to Philip regarding their right to graze their beasts peacefully in the forest of Lyons, without paying pannage or pasturage, and to have wood to burn for their house called *La Maladrerie* in the forest. John Le Veneur and the *bailli* of Gisors have been preventing Mont-aux-Malades from enjoying these rights, which has been of great detriment to the community. Therefore, Philip instructs the two men to cease from obstructing the leper house's enjoyment of these rights.

[ADSM, 25HP47(11)(xix)]

(b) 18 February 1331 (original copy in French made under the seal of obligations of the *vicomté* of Rouen), at Louvre-lès-Paris

Philip VI gives greetings to Peter de Machau and John de Bardilli, masters and inquisitors of waters and forests. The master of Salle-aux-Puelles, Rouen has made a complaint to him. It regards the fact that he and his predecessors had for a long time been in peaceful possession of 'an enclosed hedged area of ditches and planted trees', which John Le Veneur, master of the king's forests, has prevented Salle-aux-Puelles from enjoying.

[ADSM, H-Dépôt 1, A39]

77. Ralph and William d'Esneval

n.d. (c. 1174–1200; original)

Ralph and his brother William have granted in perpetual alms to Mont-aux-Malades an annual rent of 20 *sous* (10 *sous* from Ralph's mill at Sainte-Croix and 10 *sous* from William's English revenues) to be paid on the anniversary of their mother's death. If William's funds run out, Ralph will also pay his brother's contribution.

[ADSM, 25HP1(1)(viii). See also Langlois, *Histoire*, 93, 101. Two further brothers, Renaud de Pavilly and Walter, are witnesses to the charter. The fact that William d'Esneval's revenues from England are considered potentially vulnerable probably dates this act to the years immediately preceding the annexation of Normandy in 1204.]

78. Ralph the Jew

n.d. (1206–7, 1210–12 or 1213–18, original)

For the salvation of himself, his parents, ancestors, children and successors, Ralph has donated in perpetuity, to God and St Mary and St Thomas the Martyr of Mont-aux-Malades, 10 *sous* of rent due from a house in the parish of Saint-Vigor, Rouen. While Ralph is alive, Mont-aux-Malades should only receive 5 *sous* annually; after his death, it should receive the full 10 *sous*.

[ADSM, 25HP3(6)(iv). On Ralph the Jew see Brenner and Hicks, 'The Jews of Rouen', 378–9.]

79. Ralph Legoix de Montigny

The Friday before the purification of the Virgin, 1238 (act of Peter de Colle-mezzo, archbishop of Rouen, at Saint-Wandrille, copied into the thirteenth-century cartulary of the abbey of Saint-Georges de Boscherville)

The abbot and community of Saint-Georges de Boscherville have informed Peter de Collemezzo that Ralph Legoix has entered Mont-aux-Malades, donating himself and his possessions to the leper house. However, he had previously given himself and his possessions to the abbey of Saint-Georges. The abbot and community of Saint-Georges demand that Ralph should be compelled to leave Mont-aux-Malades and return with his possessions, worth 500 *livres* of Tours, to Saint-Georges. Peter de Collemezzo rules that the abbot and community should hold whatever lands and revenues Ralph had bestowed on them, and that Ralph should give them 30 *livres* of Tours. However, he does not order Ralph to return to Saint-Georges.

[BM, Rouen, MS Y52, fos 146v–147r. See Langlois, *Histoire*, 329. See also BM, Rouen, MS Y52 at fos 145r–146r (Ralph Legoix and his wife Matilda have accepted fraternity in life and death at Saint-Georges and make an alms gift to the abbey, March 1234) and fo. 146r–v (the official of Rouen confirms the alms gift of Ralph Legoix and Matilda to Saint-Georges, March 1234).]

80. Ralph, son of Stephen

February 1161 (original is undated; a slightly different version in a late thirteenth-century *vidimus* of the *vicomte* of Rouen is dated February 1161, indicating that there were at least two original versions, of which apparently only one, undated, survives)

In pure, perpetual and free alms, Ralph has donated the church of Saint-Pierre at Carville and the chapel of Saint-Ouen at Longpaon to Mont-aux-Malades. The act is ratified in the presence of 'both parishioners and others assembled in the church of Saint-Pierre [at Carville]'.

[ADSM, 25HP36 (original, late thirteenth-century *vidimus* containing the slightly different, dated version, and 1301 *vidimus* of the *vicomte* of Rouen containing the undated version); 25HP46 (seventeenth-century copy of the undated version); edited in Langlois, *Histoire*, 405. See also Langlois, *Histoire*, 15, and Farin, *Histoire*, ii/6, 30.]

81. [Renaud Barbou], *bailli* of Rouen (1275–86)

December 1283 (?eighteenth-century paper copy)

The *bailli* gives notice that, in the name of the king, he has given in perpetual farm to the mayor and citizens of Rouen various perches of land at Rouen, including the perch of the 'lepers' cabin'[22] situated at the Porte Saint-Ouen, between the city wall and the road to Saint-Nicaise, stretching from the pavement up to the wall of Saint-Ouen.

[BM, Rouen, Chartrier de la ville, tiroir 324, dossier 1. The full charter is edited in Chéruel, *Histoire*, i. 285–8. See also Chéruel, *Histoire*, ii, 'Plan de la ville de Rouen, et de ses principaux edifices jusqu'à la fin du XIVe siècle' (fold-out map engraved by A. Péron at rear of volume), showing the 'Bordellum leprosorum' just outside the Porte Saint-Ouen. For Renaud Barbou 'le Vieux', *bailli* of Rouen, see Veyrat, *Essai chronologique*, 46–9, 261.]

82. Renaud du Châtel, mayor of Rouen in 1253, Bertin du Châtel, mayor of Rouen in 1266 and Theobald du Châtel, brothers

19 June 1247 (two original copies of the same act)

Renaud, Bertin and Theobald have granted to Mont-aux-Malades the rent which their brother Robin du Châtel transferred to the leper house.

[ADSM, 25HP1(8)(iii), (v). *See* Figure 10. The name Robin, as opposed to Robert, is derived from a caption on the verso of 25HP1(8)(xxxii), which reveals that in 1242 Robin donated a rent to Mont-aux-Malades for his salvation.]

83. Richard I, king of England (1189–99)

4 April 1195 (6th year of his reign; fourteenth-century copy), at Bec-Hellouin

For the salvation of his soul and those of his father King Henry and his ancestors and successors, Richard has donated the church of (Saint-Martin du) Grand-Couronne in perpetual alms to the leprous women of Quevilly, with the things pertaining to it, all its liberties and free customs, and all its integrity.

[ADSM, 26HP7; edited in *Letters and charters of King Richard I*, 3890R (provisional number)]

84. Richard du Bosc, of the parish of Saint-Maclou, Rouen

1297 (original act in French of the *vicomte* of Rouen)

For 15 *sous* of Tours (current money) annual rent, Richard has taken in fief and perpetual hereditary possession from Mont-aux-Malades a tenement in the parish of Saint-Maclou, situated between his own tenement and the Aubette river.

[ADSM, 25HP6]

---

2 'Bordelli leprosorum', which could also mean 'lepers' brothel'.

85. Richard Marshal, later earl of Pembroke (1231–4)

May 1223 (original), at Rouen

Richard confirms the sale of a house by his man Robert Lavenier to Mont-aux-Malades. For the sake of his ancestors' souls, Richard has given to Mont-aux-Malades a pair of fur gloves which he held as rent from the house, in return for a pair of 'single gloves' to the value of 3 *deniers* (current money) to be delivered annually at Easter to himself and his heirs.

[ADSM, 25HP1(1)(ii); Power, 'French interests of the Marshal earls', 213 n. 75]

86. [Richard, prior ? –1298] and the community of Mont-aux-Malades

18 February 1297 (original)

The prior and community of Mont-aux-Malades give greetings. Following a dispute between Mont-aux-Malades and the abbey of Saint-Ouen, Rouen, regarding the provisions for leprous monks from Saint-Ouen when resident at Mont-aux-Malades, the following arrangements have been established. Each day, a monk from Saint-Ouen should receive bread and 1 gallon of wine from the abbey. He should also receive two pieces of meat (one fresh and one salted) and have five eggs or three herrings (his manservant is to enjoy three eggs or two herrings). The monk is to have a sufficient supply of salt, and to enjoy a pittance of meat, fish or wine as often as do the canons of Mont-aux-Malades, as if he is one of them. The monk is to have a candle and wood to burn as necessary, and to be allowed to return home [i.e. to Saint-Ouen] whenever he needs to. The monk's manservant is to receive 5 *sous* of Tours as payment annually from the prior of Mont-aux-Malades or his deputy. If several monks of Saint-Ouen are resident at Mont-aux-Malades at the same time, each is to receive the entitlement outlined above from the cellar and kitchen. After these monks die, all their possessions (belonging to Saint-Ouen) are to be retained by the prior of Mont-aux-Malades or his deputy until other leprous monks of Saint-Ouen come to the leper house.

[ADSM, 14H660(i). See Langlois, *Histoire*, 124–5, where it is claimed that Saint-Ouen's monks occupied a special house at Mont-aux-Malades and received certain privileges in return for Mont-aux-Malades's right to cut wood from a forest owned by Saint-Ouen, and Paul Le Cacheux, *Répertoire numérique des archives départementales antérieures à 1790: Seine-Inférieure: Archives ecclésiastiques: série H, tome IV (fascicule 1): Abbaye de Saint-Ouen de Rouen (14H1 à 14H926)*, 200–1.]

87. Richard Talbot

n.d. (probably 1166; original)

Richard confirms the sale of land and a house in the forecourt of Rouen cathedral by William and Vincent, the sons of Richard, son of Gosbert, and their sister Emma to Mont-aux-Malades for 330 marks of silver. In Richard Talbot's presence, the siblings have received part payment 'from Nicholas, prior of the lepers'. Richard has invested

Mont-aux-Malades with his own right of access to the property, and refers to his father's earlier gift of 5 *sous* (annual rent) to the leper house. Richard reserves a right to receive hospitality at the house in the forecourt of the cathedral: the guests staying there must give him warmth, shelter and the use of the utensils of the house. These provisions are granted by Richard's sons Hugh and William. The agreement is concluded in the presence of William de Malpalu, justiciar of the king.

[ADSM, 25HP1(22)(ix). See Haskins, *Norman institutions*, 326 n. 1, and Arnoux, 'Les Origines', 147. In August 1167 Prior Nicholas of Mont-aux-Malades complained to Thomas Becket of the debt that he held for a house purchased the previous year: CTB i. 622–3 (no. 132). He may well have been referring to this purchase, which would date Richard Talbot's act to 1166.]

88. Robert de Fay, of the parish of Languetot

March 1243 (original)

Robert has granted to Prior Bartholomew and the community of Mont-aux-Malades the house, enclosed land and green land which he bought from Robert de Sochons. The prior and community have given Robert de Fay 15 *livres* in recogntion of his grant, and 10 *sous* to Robert du Mont-Guérout, carpenter, who has sworn not to oppose the grant.

[ADSM, 25HP1(1)(ix)]

89. Robert Lavenier, citizen of Rouen

March 1223 (original)

With the consent of his wife Helvisia de Mara and his son Robert, cleric, Robert Lavenier has granted to Mont-aux-Malades a tenement situated in front of the forecourt of Rouen cathedral. In return, Mont-aux-Malades is to deliver a pair of gloves worth 3 *deniers* (usual money) annually at Easter to Robert and his heirs.

[ADSM, 25HP1(12)(iv)]

90. Robert Le Candelier and his wife Isabella, of the parish of Saint-Maclou, Rouen

February 1251 (original act of the official of Rouen)

Robert and Isabella have sold to Mont-aux-Malades, for 100 *sous* of Tours, 10 *sous* (usual money) annual rent due from the couple's tenement in the parish of Saint-Maclou.

[ADSM, 25HP6]

91. Robert Le Noir, his wife Basire and his mother Nicole La Forestière, of the parish of Sotteville-lès-Rouen

1297 (original act in French of the *vicomte* of Rouen)

For 8 *livres* of Tours, Robert, Basire and Nicole have sold to Mont-aux-Malades a piece of land in the parish of Sotteville-lès-Rouen, adjoining the land of Mont-aux-Malades.

[ADSM, 25HP47(15)(iii)]

92. Robert, prior of Mont-aux-Malades (1191–1218)

(a) n.d. (1191–1218; original)

Robert and the whole community of Mont-aux-Malades give notice that, in their presence, Henry de Joinville, with the consent of his wife Alix and daughter Haisia, has sold to Thomas Freschet the land which he held from Mont-aux-Malades in the parish of Saint-Jean-sur-Renelle, Rouen, for 20 *livres* of Anjou. Henry has entirely relinquished the fief to Mont-aux-Malades; the leper house community grants the land to Thomas for 10 *sous* of Anjou (usual money) annual rent. This was confirmed in the chapter at Mont-aux-Malades in the presence of all the brothers.

[ADSM, 25HP6]

(b) n.d. (1191–1218, probably 1210 ('1210' is written by later hands on the front and reverse of the charter; original)

Robert and the community of Mont-aux-Malades have granted to John d'Offranville their tenement 'on the Renelle [river]' which Robert de Saint-Jacques gave to Mont-aux-Malades.

[ASDM, 25HP1(8)(xxxiii)]

(c) n.d. (1193–4 or 1201–3; original), drawn up in the chapter of Mont-aux-Malades and confirmed before the commune of Rouen

For a lump sum of 50 *livres* of Anjou and 12 *sous* (usual money) annual rent, Robert and the community of Mont-aux-Malades, both the healthy and the sick, have granted in hereditary tenure to Ralph de Cailli [mayor of Rouen in 1198 and 1202] the tenement and houses in the rues Burnenc and Brasière, Rouen, which John Pigache gave them in perpetual alms when he took the habit at Mont-aux-Malades.

[ASDM, 25HP1(10)(xiii)]

93. Robert de Saint-Jacques and his wife Emma

n.d. (1181–2; original)

Inspired by piety, for the salvation of themselves, their ancestors and their benefactors, with the consent of their son Peter, Robert and Emma have given to Mont-aux-Malades their tenement in the alley of Saint-Patrice, Rouen, with its buildings, appendages and revenues. An annual rent of 16 *sous* (current money at Rouen) is due to the lord of the fief, at that time Stephen Clarembaud, who has consented to the gift.

[ADSM, 25HP1(8)(xiv)]

94. Roger, son of Ansger de Castenay

1 March 1220 (original charter of Robert Poulain, archbishop of Rouen)

Archbishop Robert gives notice that, in his *curia*, Roger, son of Ansger de Castenay, having decided to set out for Boulogne, has bequeathed half his house in the parish of Saint-Vincent, Rouen, to La Madeleine hospital and Mont-aux-Malades. If Roger dies in Boulogne or does not return, the two houses will possess this property in pure and perpetual alms (through the rent pertaining to it); if Roger returns, he will freely retain the property.

[ADSM, 25HP1(10)]

95. Roscelin, son of Clarembaud, Henry II's chamberlain

n.d. (1154–64; four original sheets of parchment tied together and a seventeenth-century copy of (4) only)

(1) An oration concerning Hugh of Amiens, archbishop of Rouen.

(2) Confirmation of Roscelin's act by Hugh of Amiens, describing Roscelin as 'our parishioner'.

(3) An oration for the absolution and resurrection of Roscelin's soul.

(4) Roscelin's act founding the parish church of Saint-Gilles at Mont-aux-Malades. For the remission of his sins, Roscelin grants to the church of Saint-Gilles 7 *livres* of rent in perpetual alms. He grants his house and garden by the church of Saint-Sauveur, Rouen, rent from his house in the market which Everard holds, and rent from the house Hugh Berengarius holds from him by Le Donjon. Roscelin and the prior of Mont-aux-Malades have arranged for one of the canons of Mont-aux-Malades to serve in the church of Saint-Gilles. Since he is its founder, Roscelin chooses to be buried in Saint-Gilles. He asks for Saint-Gilles to remain in being in perpetuity.

[ADSM, 25HP1(10)(xii) (original), 25HP46 (seventeenth-century copy of [4] only); edited in Langlois, *Histoire*, 398; Thomas G. Waldman, 'Hugh "of Amiens", archbishop of Rouen (1130–64)', unpubl. D.Phil diss. Oxford 1970, 330 (no. 78); Arnoux, 'Les Origines', 330–1. See also Langlois, *Histoire*, 6; Arnoux, 'Les Origines', 63, 145. Arnoux argues (p. 330) that the four sheets of parchment are later copies, but they appear to be original.]

96. Rotrou of Warwick, archbishop of Rouen (1165–84)

(a) n.d. (1165–84, probably *c.* 1165; original and seventeenth- and eighteenth-century copies)

Archbishop Rotrou confirms the rules for the annual fair at Mont-aux-Malades laid down by his predecessor Hugh of Amiens. Those who attend the fair established by Henry II, that takes place on the calends of September (1–8 September), will have one third of their penance for the relevant year remitted. If they die during the year, they will be absolved of their sins and 'will not want for care' [regarding funerary and burial services, and the care of their souls]. They will also be absolved of forgotten sins and penances. Those travelling to and from the fair do so under the protection of the Church of Rouen. Anyone who troubles them on their journey will be excommunicated until they have made amends. Rotrou orders deans and priests to receive clerics leading visitors to the fair kindly in their churches.

[ADSM, 25HP1(10)(xi) (original and eighteenth-century copy), 25HP7(xi), fo. 1r–v (seventeenth-century copy). See also Langlois, *Histoire*, 12–14.]

(b) n.d. (February 1165–73/? February 1165–March 1170 [date of Henry II's act donating the church of Nointot]; original and seventeenth-century copy)

Rotrou confirms Mont-aux-Malades's possession of the church [Saint-Sauveur] at Nointot.

[ASDM, 25HP7(viii) (original), 25HP46 (seventeenth-century copy)]

97. Silvester du Marché

(a) n.d. (1195 or 1198–1200; original and seventeenth-century copy)

For 7 *livres* of Anjou, Silvester has sold to Prior Robert of Mont-aux-Malades and the community, both the healthy and the sick, 12 *sous* of annual rent due from properties at Rouen and in the district of Bouvreuil [a suburb of Rouen]. The rent consists of 4 *sous* of Anjou from the house which Richard Maskepain holds from Silvester in the parish of Saint-Martin-sur-Renelle, Rouen, 4 *sous* from the house which Geoffrey Le Changeur holds from Silvester at Bouvreuil, and 4 *sous* from the house which William Fromont holds from Silvester at Bouvreuil.

[AN, Paris, S4889B dossier 13, nos 9 (seventeenth-century copy), 11 (original)]

(b) 1211 (original, issued before John Luce, mayor of Rouen)

For the salvation of his soul and those of his ancestors and benefactors, Silvester has donated a piece of land in the rue Wanterie [Rouen] to Mont-aux-Malades in pure and perpetual alms. The land is situated between the land of the heirs of Robert, son of Gilbert, and that of the heirs of Renaud de Castenay.

[ASDM, 25HP1(13)(ii). See Arnoux, 'Les Origines', 147–8, noting that Silvester, a wealthy burgess, was also a benefactor of Rouen's La Madeleine hospital.]

98. Simon Le Porchier, knight, Philip VI's official in charge of waters and forests

(a) 19 May 1337, at Rouen (original act in French)

John Le Veneur, knight, a previous official in charge of waters and forests, prevented Mont-aux-Malades from enjoying its right of exemption from paying pannage for its pigs in the manor of *La Maladrerie* at Lilly in the forest of Lyons. Mont-aux-Malades contested this right. John Le Veneur maintained the contrary, arguing that through certain charters and the gift of the king [Henry II], Mont-aux-Malades was exempt from paying pasturage in the forest of Lyons, but not from pannage. Simon Le Porchier confirms that, on 24 November 1334, Philip VI ruled in favour of Mont-aux-Malades.

[ASDM, 25HP47(11)(v)]

(b) 22 February 1341, issued under the seal of obligations of the *vicomté* of Rouen (original act in French)

This charter relates to the dispute in (a) above.

[ASDM, 25HP47(11)(xxv)]

99. Simon de Mara, master of arts and medicine, subdeacon of Rouen cathedral

5 February 1447 (original)

His testament. Among his bequests, he grants 30 *sous* of Tours to La Madeleine hospital, and arranges for 20 *sous* to be distributed to the poor at the hospital by his executors on the anniversary of his death. He also grants 5 *sous* of Tours 'to the lepers of the four gates of Rouen'. He asks to be buried near Guillaume Desjardins [canon of Rouen cathedral (1421–38) and master of medicine].

[ADSM, G3437. For Simon de Mara (d. 1448 at Rouen) see Wickersheimer, *Dictionnaire biographique*, 740–1, and Tabbagh, *Fasti*, 368 (no. 341)]

100. Stephen de Maromme, of the parish of Saint-Paul near Rouen

March 1253 (original act of the official of Rouen)

For 7 ½ *livres*, with the consent of his mother Helvisia and his wife Matilda, Stephen has sold to Mont-aux-Malades a piece of land and two fields at Maromme, between the land on the river bank of Mont-aux-Malades and Stephen's own land. Stephen already held this land from Mont-aux-Malades; it stretches 'up to the land of the said religious in the direction of their mill'. Mont-aux-Malades will pay 18 *deniers* of Tours annual rent to Stephen and his heirs for the land.

[ADSM, 25HP47(3)(iv)]

101. Stephen Pance de Chevire

April 1222 (original)

With the consent of his wife Haisia, Stephen has granted to Mont-aux-Malades 30 *sous* (usual money) rent due from various properties in the parish of Saint-Martin-sur-Renelle, Rouen. He and his heirs guarantee this grant in return for a pair of white gloves worth 2 *deniers*, to be delivered annually.

[ASDM, 25HP1(8)(xxvii)]

102. Walter and Robert Goobondi, brothers, and their sister Alicia, of the parishes of Déville and Maromme

March 1253 (original charter of the official of Rouen)

For 6 *livres* of Tours, with the consent of Eustacia (Walter's wife) and Basilia (Robert's wife), Walter, Robert and Alicia have sold to Mont-aux-Malades a piece of land and half a watercress bed in the parish of Déville. Mont-aux-Malades will pay 1 ounce of cumin annual rent to the three siblings for this land.

[ADSM, 25HP47(3)(ii)]

103. Walter Le Blanc and his wife Nicola of the parish of Saint-Jean-sur-Renelle, Rouen

1247 (original charter of the official of Rouen)

For 50 *livres* of Tours, Walter and Nicola have taken in fief and hereditary possession from Mont-aux-Malades a tenement in the parish of Saint-Martin-sur-Renelle, Rouen. This tenement was granted by William Le Tort (Bouglarius) and his wife Alicia to Mont-aux-Malades for their salvation in pure and perpetual alms. It is situated next to Walter and Nicola's house, for which they already pay 10 *sous* annual rent to Mont-aux-Malades. Walter and Nicola and their heirs are to pay 30 *sous* annual rent to Mont-aux-Malades for the tenement.

[ADSM, 25HP1(8)(xxiii)]

104. William, younger brother of Henry II (born July 1136, d. 29 January 1164)

n.d. (July 1158–29 January 1164; copy made in 1674 of King Henry v's 3 January 1420 *vidimus* of William's act)

For the salvation of himself, his ancestors and his brother Geoffrey [who died on 26 July 1158], Prince William donates 40 *sous* annual rent to Mont-aux-Malades from his revenues at Dieppe. [His mother the Empress Matilda is the first witness of his act.]

[AN, Paris, S4889B, liasse 1, no. 7 (1674 copy of Henry v's 3 January 1420 *vidimus* of four twelfth-century acts relating to Mont-aux-Malades, the third of which is William's donation), fo. 1v]

105. William Baril

n.d. (1130–64, probably *c.* 1140–64, in an original confirmation by Hugh of Amiens, archbishop of Rouen and a seventeenth-century copy)

William has given to the lepers of Mont-aux-Malades his land of Le Mont-Robert, in fief and hereditary possession, in return for 1 pound of pepper annually (for William and his heirs). In return for this donation, the lepers have given William 32 marks of silver: 20 marks for Laurence, son of Ralph, son of Robert, for consenting to the transaction, and 12 marks for William himself.

[ADSM, 25HP10(xxii) (original); AN, Paris, S4889B, liasse 1, no. 1, fo. 1r–v (seventeenth-century copy). See Langlois, *Histoire*, 16.]

106. William de la Barre

n.d. (1206–7, 1210–12 or 1213–18 [drawn up before John Luce, mayor of Rouen]; original)

For 21 *livres* of Tours, William has sold to Mont-aux-Malades a total of 39 *sous* annual rent due from various individuals and relating to various lands and properties in and around Rouen.

[ADSM, 25HP1(8)(ii)]

107. William, son of Bartholomew de Grand-Pont

n.d. (1195 or 1198–1200 [drawn up before Matthew Le Gros, mayor of Rouen]; original)

William has donated to the lepers and brothers of Mont-aux-Malades his interests in the fief that Guy Crostele held from him in [the rue] Wanterie, with the revenues he held from the fief (22 *sous* annual rent on the feast of St Michael, and 1 *quartarium* of pork and 1 pint of wine at Christmas). The lepers will hold the fief and all things pertaining to it in free, pure and perpetual alms. In return, the lepers have recieved William in the habit of their religion. Geoffrey de Val-Richer, Clarembaud Le Roux, Ralph Amiot and Ralph the Jew are among the witnesses to the charter.

[AN, Paris, S4889B, dossier 13, no. 12]

108. William de Beuzeville, knight

December (the octave of St Andrew) 1225 (original)

For his salvation and that of all his ancestors and successors, William has donated to Mont-aux-Malades the land that William Lescolier held from him, in pure and perpetual alms [the location of the land is not specified].

[ASDM, 25HP1(1)(v)]

109. William L'Aiguillon, knight, son of William de Mortagne

(a) n.d. (*c.* 1174–90; original)

With the consent of his wife Sybil, William has granted the sale of land by Warner Escalope to Prior Herbert and the brothers of Mont-aux-Malades. Warner was paid 6 *livres* of Anjou for the land. William has received a silver wine cup from Mont-aux-Malades in return for granting the sale. William has also granted that Mont-aux-Malades should hold the land in pure and perpetual alms without owing any lay service, excepting 2 *sous* which are to be returned annually to William and his heirs.

[ASDM, 25HP10]

(b) n.d. (*c.* 1174–1200; in an original *vidimus* of the *vicomte* of Rouen, dated 1301, and a seventeenth-century copy)

With the consent of his wife Sybil, William has donated the church of Saint-Aubin-de-Beuzeville-la-Vaveske [Beuzevillette] to Mont-aux-Malades in pure and perpetual alms.

[ADSM, 25HP39 (original *vidimus*), 25HP46 (seventeenth-century copy); edited in Langlois, *Histoire*, 429–30. See also Langlois, *Histoire*, 87, and Farin, *Histoire*, ii/6, 30.]

110. William L'Aiguillon, knight, son of William L'Aiguillon and Sybil

March 1228 (notification by Theobald of Amiens, archbishop of Rouen, in an original *vidimus* of the *vicomte* of Rouen, 1301)

For the salvation of himself, his wife and his sons, William confirms his father's gift of the church of Saint-Aubin-de-Beuzeville-la-Vaveske (Beuzevillette) to Mont-aux-Malades. For 2 *sous* annual rent, he also confirms the sale of land by Warner Escalope to Mont-aux-Malades.

[ADSM, 25HP39]

111. William Le Moine and his sister Maria (the wife of John Leporis), of the parish of Déville

March 1253 (original charter of the official of Rouen)

For 40 *sous* of Tours, with the consent of John Leporis, William and Maria have sold to Mont-aux-Malades a piece of land in the parish of Déville near the springs of Mont-aux-Malades. The leper house will pay 1 ounce of cumin as annual rent to William, Maria and their heirs for the land.

[ADSM, 25HP47(3)(vi)]

112. William Le Tort Bouglarius and his wife Alicia

September 1233 (original charter of the official of Rouen)

For their salvation and that of their ancestors, William and Alicia have donated in pure and perpetual alms to Mont-aux-Malades a house with attached land in the parish of Saint-Martin-sur-Renelle, Rouen, which they already hold from Mont-aux-Malades in hereditary possession. They have also donated 3 *sous* of annual rent due from the hall of the Cordeliers adjacent to the property. William and Alicia may remain living in the property for as long as they both live.

[ADSM, 25HP1(8)(xxiv)]

113. William de Malpalu, royal justice (c. 1171–90)

n.d. (1176, 1177, 1179, 1180, 1182 or 1190 [from c. 1174; witnessed by Bartholomew Fergant as mayor of Rouen], in an original *vidimus* of the *vicomte* of Rouen, 1301, also containing the charter of Florent de Grémonville)

For his salvation and that of his ancestors, William has given in perpetual alms to the lepers of Mont-Rouen the land and two hosts at Mont de la Coudre which he held from Florent de Grémonville in hereditary fief, excepting the sum of 13 *sous* (usual money) annual rent that he paid to Florent.

[ADSM, 25HP1(2)(i). See Langlois, *Histoire*, 87. On William de Malpalu see Veyrat, *Essai chronologique*, 19–20, 261.]

114. William de Milloel

1252 (original act of the official of Rouen)

In return for 100 *sous* of Tours, William Le Sochon and his siblings Ansquetillus, Sanson and Lucia have ratified the gift by their brother William de Milloel, formerly clerk of Stephen de la Porte, knight, *bailli* of Rouen, to Mont-aux-Malades. In his final testament, for the salvation of his soul, William de Milloel donated his tenement in the parish of Saint-Laurent, Rouen to the leper house.

[ADSM, 25HP1(17)(xiii). For Stephen de la Porte, *bailli* of Rouen (1247–54) see Veyrat, *Essai chronologique*, 38–9, 261, and Strayer, *The administration of Normandy*, 96, 97, 110.]

115. William, prior of Mont-aux-Malades (1222–33)

May 1233 (original)

For 24 *livres* of Tours, William and the whole community, both healthy and leprous, have granted to William Peteum, citizen of Rouen, and his wife Matilda a tenement of wood and stone, with its cellar, in the parish of Saint-Sauveur in Rouen's market. The tenement is situated close to the land of Walter de Saint-Léonard, Clarembaud Le Roux and Ralph de Boes [mayor of Rouen, 1223–4]. William Peteum and his wife are to pay 14 *livres* (usual money at Rouen) annual rent for the tenement to Mont-aux-Malades.

[ADSM, 25HP1(10)(ii)]

116. William Tocqueville

April 1270 (original)

For 12 *livres* of Tours, William has sold to Nicholas Pigache, chaplain of Mont-aux-Malades, a garden and piece of land in the parish of Saint-Aignan. These are to be held by Nicholas and his heirs, in return for 6 *sous*, 6 *deniers* annual rent.

[ADSM, 25HP1(6)]

Bibliography

Unpublished primary sources

London, British Library
MS Add. Charter 11522 Confirmation by Henry II of a grant to Mont-aux-Malades by Osbert, lord of Préaux, undated (1156–Apr. 1166/ ?May 1165, in a *vidimus* of Pierre du Busc, keeper of the seal of obligations of the *vicomté* of Rouen, 30 Aug. 1424

London, Wellcome Library
MS 130 Bernard de Gordon, *Practica medicinalis (Lilium medicinae)*, fourteenth century
MS 5133/1 Agreement issued by Simon Paine, mayor of Pontoise, for the admission of Jehan Duquesnoy called 'le Bourgignon' to the *leprosarium* of Saint-Lazare at Aumône near Pontoise, 17 May 1412

Paris, Archives Nationales
*K23 nos 15 22, 15 22b Grant of Geoffrey of Anjou in favour of the lepers of Rouen, n.d. (1145–50) Original charter and *vidimus* issued by the *vicomté* of Rouen, 28 Dec. 1437
S4889B, S4929–30, dossier 6 Documents relating to Mont-aux-Malades

Rouen, Archives départementales de Seine-Maritime
Archives de la Ville, déliberations, registre A4 Medieval municipal archives of Rouen
G1236 Testament of John Hardi, 1304, in a *vidimus* of the official of Rouen, 1353
G2140 Register of Rouen cathedral chapter, 6 Sept. 1476–31 Dec. 1479
G6606 Documents regarding suspected cases of leprosy in the parish of Saint-Gervais, Rouen, 1535–40
G6897 Register of accounts of the parish of Saint-Maclou, Rouen, Christmas 1585–Christmas 1586
G6898 Register of accounts of the parish of Saint-Maclou, Rouen, Christmas 1589–Christmas 1590
G6902 Register of accounts of the parish of Saint-Maclou, Rouen, 1591
G7137 Testament of John Hardi, 1304, in a *vidimus* of the official of Rouen, 1304, Friday after the commission of St Paul the Apostle
H-Dépôt 1, A39, F1 Documents relating to Salle-aux-Puelles and La Madeleine hospital
14H Archive of the abbey of Saint-Ouen, Rouen
25HP Archive of Mont-aux-Malades, Rouen
26HP Archive of the priory of Saint-Lô, Rouen
27HP Archive of the abbey of La Trinité-du-Mont, Rouen

55H Archive of the abbey of Saint-Amand, Rouen

Rouen, Bibliothèque municipale
MS Y42 Fifteenth-century memorial book of La Madeleine hospital, Rouen
MS Y52 Thirteenth-century cartulary of the abbey of Saint-Georges-de-Boscher-
ville
Tiroirs 109, 324 Medieval municipal archives of Rouen

**Rouen, Direction Régionale des Affaires Culturelles de Haute-
Normandie/Service Régional de l'Inventaire Général**
Dossier 76 INV 527 File on the commune of Mont-Saint-Aignan

Published primary sources

*Cartulaire de la léproserie du Grand-Beaulieu et du prieuré de Notre-Dame de la
Bourdinière*, ed. René Merlet and Maurice Jusselin, Chartres 1909
Cartulaire normand de Philippe-Auguste, Louis VIII, Saint-Louis et Philippe-le-Hardi,
ed. Léopold Delisle, Caen 1852, repr. Geneva 1978
Catalogue des actes de Philippe-Auguste, ed. Léopold Delisle, Paris 1856
*Un Censier normand du XIIIe siècle: le Livre des Jurés de l'abbaye Saint-Ouen de
Rouen*, ed. Denise Angers, Catherine Bébéar and Henri Dubois, Paris 2001
Chronique normande de Pierre Cochon, notaire apostolique à Rouen, ed. Charles de
Robillard de Beaurepaire, Rouen 1870
Chronique de Robert de Torigni, abbé du Mont-Saint-Michel, ed. Léopold Delisle,
Rouen 1872–3
Concilia Rotomagensis provinciae, ed. Guillaume Bessin, Rouen 1717
The correspondence of Thomas Becket, archbishop of Canterbury, 1162–1170, ed.
and trans. Anne J. Duggan, Oxford 2000
Decrees of the ecumenical councils, ed. and trans. Norman P. Tanner, London 1990
Documents concernant les pauvres de Rouen: extraits des archives de l'Hôtel-de-Ville,
ed. G. Panel, Rouen 1917–19
'The "Draco Normannicus" of Etienne of Rouen', in *Chronicles of the reigns
of Stephen, Henry II and Richard I*, ii, ed. Richard Howlett, London 1885,
589–781
The Ecclesiastical history of Orderic Vitalis, ed. and trans. Marjorie Chibnall,
Oxford 1969–80
*The 'Gesta normannorum ducum' of William of Jumièges, Orderic Vitalis, and Robert
of Torigni*, ed. and trans. Elisabeth van Houts, Oxford 1992–5
Gordon, Bernard de, *Practica seu Lilium medicinae*, Naples 1480
Haskins, Charles Homer, *Norman institutions*, Cambridge, MA 1918
The Holy Bible, containing the Old and New Testaments, authorised King James
version, London n.d.
Honorii III Romani pontificis opera omnia, ed. C. Horoy, Paris 1879–80
*The letters and charters of Gilbert Foliot, abbot of Gloucester (1139–48), bishop of
Hereford (1148–63) and London (1163–87)*, ed. Adrian Morey and C. N. L.
Brooke, Cambridge 1967

The letters and charters of King Henry II (1154–1189), ed. Nicholas Vincent and others, Oxford forthcoming

The letters and charters of King Richard I (1189–1199), ed. Judith Everard and Nicholas Vincent, Oxford forthcoming

The letters of John of Salisbury, II: The later letters (1163–1180), ed. and trans. W. J. Millor and C. N. L. Brooke, Oxford 1979

Materials for the history of Thomas Becket, archbishop of Canterbury, ed. J. C. Robertson (Rolls Series, 1875–85)

'Miracula, quae Rothomagi in Normannia ab anno Christi MCCLXI usque ad annum MCCLXX contigerunt', in *Acta Sanctorum Augusti*, i, Antwerp 1733, repr. Brussels 1970, 648–56

Normanniae nova chronica ab anno Christi CCCCLXXIII. ad annum MCCCLXX-VIII: e tribus chronicis mss: Sancti Laudi, Sanctae Catharinae et Majoris Ecclesiae Rotomagensium collecta, ed. A. Chéruel, Caen 1850

L'Obituaire de l'Hôpital des Quinze-Vingts de Paris, ed. Jean-Loup Lemaître, Paris 2011

Ordonnances des rois de France de la troisième race, xx, ed. Claude de Pastoret, Paris 1840

Pipe rolls of the Exchequer of Normandy for the reign of Henry II, 1180 and 1184, ed. Vincent Moss, London 2004

Pouillés de la province de Rouen, ed. Auguste Longnon, Paris 1903

Recueil des actes de Henri II, roi d'Angleterre et duc de Normandie, ed. Léopold Delisle and Élie Berger, Paris 1909–27

Recueil des actes de Philippe Auguste, roi de France, ed. H.-François Delaborde and others, Paris 1916–2005

Recueil d'actes de Saint-Lazare de Paris, 1124–1254, ed. Simone Lefèvre, under the direction of Lucie Fossier, Paris 2005

Recueil des historiens des Gaules et de la France, xxiii, ed. J. N. de Wailly, L. V. Delisle and C. M. G. B. Jourdain, Paris 1876

Regesta regum Anglo-Normannorum, 1066–1154, ed. H. A. Cronne, R. H. C. Davis and others, Oxford 1913–69

Regestrum visitationum archiepiscopi Rothomagensis: journal des visites pastorales d'Eude Rigaud, archevêque de Rouen. MCCXLVIII–MCCLXIX, ed. Théodose Bonnin, Rouen 1852

The register of Eudes of Rouen, trans. Sydney M. Brown and ed. Jeremiah F. O'Sullivan, New York 1964

Les Registres de Philippe Auguste, I: Texte, ed. John W. Baldwin, Paris 1992

Répertoire des documents nécrologiques français, ed. Jean-Loup Lemaître, Paris 1980–7

Répertoire des documents nécrologiques français: troisième supplément (1993–2008), ed. Jean-Loup Lemaître, Paris 2008

Rotuli chartarum in turri Londinensi asservati, I/1: (1199–1216), ed. T. Hardy, London 1837

'The Rule of Augustine (masculine version)', in *The Rule of Saint Augustine*, ed. Tarsicius J. van Bavel, and trans. Raymond Canning, Kalamazoo 1996, 11–24

Sacrorum conciliorum nova, et amplissima collectio …, xxii, ed. J. D. Mansi, Venice 1778

Statuts d'Hôtels-Dieu et de léproseries: recueil de textes du XIIe au XIVe siècle, ed. Léon Le Grand, Paris 1901

The trial of Joan of Arc, trans. and intro. Daniel Hobbins, Cambridge, MA 2005

Secondary works

Arnoux, Mathieu, 'Introduction', in Arnoux, Des Clercs, 5–9

—— 'Les Origines et le développement du mouvement canonial en Normandie', in Arnoux, Des Clercs, 11–172

—— (ed.), Des Clercs au service de la réforme: études et documents sur les chanoines réguliers de la province de Rouen, Turnhout 2000

Avril, Jean, 'Le IIIe Concile du Latran et les communautés de lépreux', Revue Mabillon lx (1981), 21–76

Baldwin, John W., The government of Philip Augustus: foundations of French royal power in the Middle Ages, Berkeley 1986

Barber, Malcolm, 'Lepers, Jews and Moslems: the plot to overthrow Christendom in 1321', History lxvi (1981), 1–17

Barlow, Frank, Thomas Becket, London 1986, repr. London 2000

Bates, David, 'Rouen from 900 to 1204: from Scandinavian settlement to Angevin "capital"', in Stratford, Medieval art, architecture and archaeology, 1–11

Beaurepaire, Charles de Robillard de, Inventaire-Sommaire des Archives départementales antérieures à 1790: Seine-Inférieure, archives ecclésiastiques – Série G, v (nos 6221–7370), Rouen 1892

Bériac, Françoise, Histoire des lépreux au moyen âge: une société d'exclus, Paris 1988

—— Des lépreux aux cagots: recherches sur les sociétés marginales en Aquitaine médiévale, Bordeaux 1990

Bériou, Nicole, 'Les Lépreux sous le regard des prédicateurs d'après les collections de sermons ad status du XIIIème siècle', in Bériou and Touati, Voluntate dei leprosus, 33–80

—— and François-Olivier Touati, Voluntate dei leprosus: les lépreux entre conversion et exclusion aux XIIème et XIIIème siècles, Spoleto 1991

Bird, J., 'Medicine for body and soul: Jacques de Vitry's sermons to hospitallers and their charges', in P. Biller and J. Ziegler (eds), Religion and medicine in the Middle Ages, York 2001, 91–108

Boeckl, Christine M., Images of leprosy: disease, religion, and politics in European art, Kirksville, MO 2011

Boldsen, Jesper L., 'Epidemiological approach to the paleopathological diagnosis of leprosy', American Journal of Physical Anthropology cxv (2001), 380–7

Bonnin, Luc, 'Saint-Thomas d'Aizier: un exemple de projet de valorisation d'un site archéologique de léproserie médiévale', in Tabuteau, Étude des lépreux, 35–6

Borradori, Piera, Mourir au monde: les lépreux dans le Pays de Vaud (XIIIe–XVIIe siècle), Lausanne 1992

Bouet, Pierre and François Neveux (eds), Les Villes normandes au moyen âge: renaissance, essor, crise: actes du colloque international de Cerisy-la-Salle (8–12 octobre 2003), Caen 2006

Boulanger, Marc, *Les Hôpitaux de Rouen: une longue et attachante histoire: des origines à nos jours*, Luneray 1988

Bourgeois, Albert, *Lépreux et maladreries du Pas-de-Calais (Xe–XVIIIe siècles)*, Arras 1972

Bowers, Barbara S. (ed.), *The medieval hospital and medical practice*, Aldershot 2007

Brenner, Elma, 'The leper house of Mont-aux-Malades, Rouen, in the twelfth and thirteenth centuries (with annexes by Bruno Tabuteau)', in Tabuteau, *Étude des lépreux*, 219–46

—— 'Recent perspectives on leprosy in medieval Western Europe', *History Compass* viii (2010), 388–406

—— 'Leprosy and public health in late medieval Rouen', in Clark and Rawcliffe, *The fifteenth century*, xii. 123–38

—— 'The care of the sick and needy in twelfth- and thirteenth-century Rouen', in Hicks and Brenner, *Society and culture*, 339–67

—— and Leonie V. Hicks, 'The Jews of Rouen in the eleventh to the thirteenth centuries', in Hicks and Brenner, *Society and culture*, 369–82

—— and Bruno Tabuteau, 'La Salle-aux-Puelles, à Rouen: une léproserie de femmes', in Bruno Tabuteau (ed.), *Les Léproseries organisées au moyen âge*, *Revue de la Société Française d'Histoire des Hôpitaux* clii (2014), 44–50

—— 'Marginal bodies and minds: responses to leprosy and mental disorders in late medieval Normandy', in Andrew Spicer and Jane Stevens Crawshaw (eds), *The problem and place of the social margins, 1300–1800*, London forthcoming

—— Meredith Cohen and Mary Franklin-Brown (eds), *Memory and commemoration in medieval culture*, Farnham 2013

Brodman, James W., *Charity and welfare: hospitals and the poor in medieval Catalonia*, Philadelphia 1998

—— 'Shelter and segregation: lepers in medieval Catalonia', in Donald J. Kagay and Theresa M. Vann (eds), *On the social origins of medieval institutions: essays in honor of Joseph F. O'Callaghan*, Leiden 1998, 35–45

—— *Charity and religion in medieval Europe*, Washington, DC 2009

Brody, Saul N., *The disease of the soul: leprosy in medieval literature*, Ithaca, NY 1974

Burckard, François, *Guide des archives de la Seine-Maritime*, I: *Généralités: archives antérieures à 1790*, Rouen 1990

Bynum, Caroline Walker, *Holy feast and holy fast: the religious significance of food to medieval women*, Berkeley 1987

Cassidy-Welch, Megan, *Imprisonment in the medieval religious imagination, c. 1150–1400*, Basingstoke 2011

Chéruel, A., *Histoire de Rouen pendant l'époque communale, 1150–1382*, Rouen 1843–4

Chibnall, Marjorie, *The Empress Matilda: queen consort, queen mother and lady of the English*, Oxford 1991

Clark, Linda and Carole Rawcliffe (eds), *The fifteenth century*, XII: *Society in an age of plague*, Woodbridge 2013

Colvin, Howard, 'The origin of chantries', *Journal of Medieval History* xxvi (2000), 163–73

Cordonnier, Mathilde, 'L'Église, les fidèles et la mort, à travers des miracles de Saint Dominique (Rouen, 1261–1270)', *Tabularia 'Études'* viii (2008), 45–57

Cottineau, L. H., *Répertoire topo-bibliographique des abbayes et prieurés*, Mâcon 1935–70

Crouch, David, 'The origin of chantries: some further Anglo-Norman evidence', *Journal of Medieval History* xxvii (2001), 159–80

Curry, Anne, 'Les Villes normandes et l'occupation anglaise: l'importance du siège de Rouen (1418–1419)', in Bouet and Neveux, *Les Villes normandes*, 109–23

Davis, Adam J., *The holy bureaucrat: Eudes Rigaud and religious reform in thirteenth-century Normandy*, Ithaca, NY 2006

Deck, Suzanne, 'Les Marchands de Rouen sous les ducs', *AN* vi (1956), 245–54

Delanes, Sabine, 'L'Aître Saint-Maclou', in Christiane Decaëns, Henry Decaëns, Jérôme Decoux and Sabine Delanes, *L'Église et l'aître Saint-Maclou, Rouen, Haute-Normandie*, [Rouen] 2012, 53–71

Delsalle, Lucien René, *Rouen et les Rouennais au temps de Jeanne d'Arc, 1400–1470*, Rouen 1982

Demaitre, Luke, 'The description and diagnosis of leprosy by fourteenth-century physicians', *Bulletin of the History of Medicine* lix (1985), 327–44

—— 'The relevance of futility: Jordanus de Turre (fl. 1313–1335) on the treatment of leprosy', *Bulletin of the History of Medicine* lxx (1996), 25–61

—— *Leprosy in premodern medicine: a malady of the whole body*, Baltimore 2007

—— *Medieval medicine: the art of healing, from head to toe*, Santa Barbara, CA 2013

Deschamps, Philippe, 'Léproseries et maladreries rouennaises: le prieuré du Mont-aux-Malades et ses rapports avec Thomas Becket', *Revue des Sociétés Savantes de Haute-Normandie* xlviii (1967), 31–46

—— 'L'Abbé Cochet, l'abbé Langlois et la formation archéologique du clergé diocésain au XIXe siècle', in *Centenaire de l'abbé Cochet 1975: actes du colloque international d'archéologie, Rouen 3-4-5 juillet 1975*, Rouen 1978, i. 29–36

Doquang, Mailan S., 'Status and the soul: commemoration and intercession in the Rayonnant chapels of northern France in the thirteenth and fourteenth centuries', in Brenner, Cohen and Franklin-Brown, *Memory and commemoration*, 93–118

Du Plessis, M. Toussaint C., *Description géographique et historique de la Haute Normandie*, Paris 1740, repr. Brionne 1971

Duchemin, P., *Petit-Quevilly et le prieuré de Saint-Julien*, Pont-Audemer 1890, repr. Saint-Étienne-du-Rouvray 1987

—— *Sotteville-lès-Rouen, et le faubourg de Saint-Sever*, Rouen 1893, repr. Paris 1990

Dugdale, William, *Monasticon anglicanum*, London 1817–30

Dumas, Geneviève, *Santé et société à Montpellier à la fin du moyen âge*, Leiden 2015

—— 'Bien public et pratiques de la santé à Montpellier au XVe siècle', in *Actes du colloque Montpellier au moyen âge: bilan et approches nouvelles, les 14 et 15 novembre 2013, Université Montpellier 3*, forthcoming

Étienne-Steiner, Claire, *La Chapelle Saint-Julien du Petit-Quevilly*, Rouen 1991

Farin, François, *Histoire de la ville de Rouen: divisée en six parties*, 3rd edn, Rouen 1731

Farmer, David H., *The Oxford dictionary of saints*, 5th edn, Oxford 2003

Farmer, Sharon, *Surviving poverty in medieval Paris: gender, ideology and the daily lives of the poor*, Ithaca, NY 2002

Fenton, Kirsten A., 'Women, property, and power: some examples from eleventh-century Rouen cartularies', in Hicks and Brenner, *Society and culture*, 227–46

Finucane, Ronald C., *Miracles and pilgrims: popular beliefs in medieval England*, London 1977, rev. Basingstoke 1995

Foreville, Raymonde, 'Les Origines normandes de la famille Becket et le culte de saint Thomas en Normandie', *Mélanges offerts à Pierre Andrieu-Guitrancourt*, *L'Année canonique* xvii (1973), 433–79

Fournée, Jean, 'Les Normands face à la peste', *Le Pays bas-normand* cxlix (1978)

—— 'Les Maladreries et les vocables de leurs chapelles', *Lèpre et lépreux en Normandie*, *Cahiers Léopold Delisle* xlvi (1997), 49–142

Gauthiez, Bernard, 'Les Maisons de Rouen, xiie–xviiie siècles', *Archéologie Médiévale* xxiii (1993), 131–217

—— 'Paris, un Rouen capétien? (Développements comparés de Rouen et Paris sous les règnes de Henri ii et Philippe Auguste)', *ANS* xvi (1993), 117–36

—— 'The urban development of Rouen, 989–1345', in Hicks and Brenner, *Society and culture*, 17–64

Geary, Patrick J., *Furta sacra: thefts of relics in the central Middle Ages*, revised edn, Princeton, NJ 1990

Geltner, Guy, *The medieval prison: a social history*, Princeton, NJ 2008

Geremek, Bronislaw, *The margins of society in late medieval Paris*, trans. J. Birrell, Cambridge 1987

—— *Poverty: a history*, trans. A. Kolakowska, Oxford 1994

Getz, Faye, *Medicine in the English Middle Ages*, Princeton, NJ 1998

Gilchrist, Roberta, *Medieval life: archaeology and the life course*, Woodbridge 2012

Giry, A., *Les Établissements de Rouen: études sur l'histoire des institutions municipales de Rouen, Falaise, Pont-Audemer, etc.*, Paris 1883–5

Glanville, Léonce de, *Histoire du prieuré de Saint-Lô de Rouen*, Rouen 1890–1

Golb, Norman, *Les Juifs de Rouen au moyen âge: portrait d'une culture oubliée*, Rouen 1985

—— *The Jews in medieval Normandy: a social and intellectual history*, Cambridge 1998

Grant, Lindy, 'Le Patronage architectural d'Henri ii et de son entourage', *Cahiers de Civilisation Médiévale* Xe–XIIe siècles xxxvii (1994), 73–84 and plates

—— *Architecture and society in Normandy, 1120–1270*, New Haven 2005

Green, Monica H., *Making women's medicine masculine: the rise of male authority in pre-modern gynaecology*, Oxford 2008

Hallam, Elizabeth M., 'Henry ii as a founder of monasteries', *Journal of Ecclesiastical History* xxviii (1977), 113–32

Harvey, Barbara, *Living and dying in England, 1100–1540: the monastic experience*, Oxford 1993

Henderson, John, *Piety and charity in late medieval Florence*, Oxford 1994

—— *The Renaissance hospital: healing the body and healing the soul*, New Haven 2006

Herval, René, *Histoire de Rouen*, Rouen 1947–9

Hicks, Leonie V., 'Exclusion as exile: spiritual punishment and physical illness in Normandy c. 1050–1300', in Laura Napran and Elisabeth van Houts (eds), *Exile in the Middle Ages: selected proceedings from the International Medieval Congress, University of Leeds, 8–11 July 2002*, Turnhout 2004, 145–58

—— *Religious life in Normandy, 1050–1300: space, gender and social pressure*, Woodbridge 2007

—— and Elma Brenner (eds), *Society and culture in medieval Rouen, 911–1300*, Turnhout 2013

Hill, Carole, *Women and religion in late medieval Norwich*, Woodbridge 2010

Honeybourne, Marjorie B., 'The leper hospitals of the London area, with an appendix on some other mediaeval hospitals of Middlesex', *Transactions of the London & Middlesex Archaeological Society* xxi (1963), 1–64

Horden, Peregrine, 'A non-natural environment: medicine without doctors and the medieval European hospital', in Bowers, *The medieval hospital*, 133–45

Howell, Martha C., 'Fixing movables: gifts by testament in late medieval Douai', *Past & Present* cl (1996), 3–45

Hue, François, *La Communauté des chirurgiens de Rouen: chirurgiens – barbiers-chirurgiens – Collège de Chirurgie, 1407–1791*, Rouen 1913

Huneycutt, Lois L., *Matilda of Scotland: a study in medieval queenship*, Woodbridge 2003

Iogna-Prat, Dominique, *Ordonner et exclure: Cluny et la société chrétienne face à l'hérésie, au judaïsme et à l'islam*, Paris 1998

Jacquart, Danielle, *Le Milieu médical en France du XIIe au XVe siècle*, Geneva 1981

—— and Claude Thomasset, *Sexuality and medicine in the Middle Ages*, trans. Matthew Adamson, Cambridge 1988

Jamroziak, Emilia, *Rievaulx abbey and its social context, 1132–1300: memory, locality, and networks*, Turnhout 2005

Jeanne, Damien, 'Quelles Problématiques pour la mort du lépreux? Sondages archéologiques du cimetière de Saint-Nicolas-de-la-Chesnaie – Bayeux', *AN* xlvii (1997), 69–90

Joanne, Adolphe, *Géographie du département de la Seine-Inférieure*, Paris 1873, repr. Évreux 1994

Johnson, Penelope D., *Equal in monastic profession: religious women in medieval France*, Chicago 1991

Kealey, Edward J., *Medieval medicus: a social history of Anglo-Norman medicine*, Baltimore 1981

Kemp, Brian, 'Maiden Bradley priory, Wiltshire, and Kidderminster church, Worcestershire', in Malcolm Barber, Patricia McNulty and Peter Noble (eds), *East Anglian and other studies presented to Barbara Dodwell, Reading Medieval Studies* xi (1985), 87–120

Kinzelbach, Annemarie, 'Infection, contagion, and public health in late medieval and early modern German imperial towns', *Journal of the History of Medicine and Allied Sciences* lxi (2006), 369–89

Lanfry, Georges, 'L'Église Saint-Jacques du Mont-aux-Malades: bref résumé d'histoire', *Bulletin de la Commission des Antiquités de la Seine Maritime* xxvii (1968–9), 167–70

Langlois, Pierre, *Histoire du prieuré du Mont-aux-Malades-lès-Rouen, et correspondance du prieur de ce monastère avec saint Thomas de Cantorbéry, 1120–1820*, Rouen 1851

Lardin, Philippe, 'Les Rouennais et la pollution à la fin du moyen âge', in Élisabeth Lalou, Bruno Lepeuple and Jean-Louis Roch (eds), *Des Châteaux et des sources: archéologie et histoire dans la Normandie médiévale: mélanges en l'honneur d'Anne-Marie Flambard Héricher*, Mont-Saint-Aignan 2008, 399–427

Le Cacheux, Marie-Josèphe, *Histoire de l'abbaye de Saint-Amand de Rouen, des origines à la fin du XVIe siècle*, Caen 1937

Le Cacheux, Paul, *Répertoire numérique des archives départementales antérieures à 1790: Seine-Inférieure: Archives ecclésiastiques: série H, tome IV (fascicule 1): Abbaye de Saint-Ouen de Rouen (14H1 à 14H926)*, Rouen 1938

Lee, Frances and John Magilton, 'Discussion', in Magilton, Lee and Boylston, *'Lepers outside the gate'*, 263–9

—— and Keith Manchester, 'Leprosy: a review of the evidence in the Chichester sample', in Magilton, Lee and Boylston, *'Lepers outside the gate'*, 208–17

Lee, Gerard A., *Leper hospitals in medieval Ireland: with a short account of the military and Hospitaller order of St Lazarus of Jerusalem*, Blackrock, Co. Dublin 1996

Lemoine, François, and Jacques Tanguy, *Rouen aux 100 clochers: dictionnaire des églises et chapelles de Rouen (avant 1789)*, Rouen 2004

Lester, Anne E., *Creating Cistercian nuns: the women's religious movement and its reform in thirteenth-century Champagne*, Ithaca, NY 2011

Lewis, Mary E., 'Infant and childhood leprosy: present and past', in Charlotte A. Roberts, Mary E. Lewis and Keith Manchester (eds), *The past and present of leprosy: archaeological, historical, palaeopathological and clinical approaches*, Oxford 2002, 163–70

Little, Lester K., *Religious poverty and the profit economy in medieval Europe*, London 1978

Lot, Ferdinand, *Études critiques sur l'abbaye de Saint-Wandrille*, Paris 1913

Mackay, Dorothy-Louise, *Les Hôpitaux et la charité à Paris au XIIIe siècle*, Paris 1923

Madeline, Fanny, 'Rouen and its place in the building policy of the Angevin kings', in Hicks and Brenner, *Society and culture*, 65–99

Magilton, John, 'The hospital of St James and St Mary Magdalene, Chichester, and other leper houses', in Bruno Tabuteau (ed.), *Lépreux et sociabilité du moyen âge aux temps modernes*, Rouen 2000, 81–91

——'The cemetery', in Magilton, Lee and Boylston, *'Lepers outside the gate'*, 84–132

——Frances Lee and Anthea Boylston (eds), *'Lepers outside the gate': excavations at the cemetery of the hospital of St James and St Mary Magdalene, Chichester, 1986–87 and 1993*, York 2008

Marcombe, David, *Leper knights: the Order of St Lazarus of Jerusalem in England, 1150–1544*, Woodbridge 2003

Marcovitch, Harvey (ed.), *Black's medical dictionary*, 41st edn, London 2005

Mesmin, Simone C., 'Waleran, count of Meulan and the leper hospital of S. Gilles de Pont-Audemer', *AN* xxxii (1982), 3–19

—— 'Du Comte à la commune: la léproserie de Saint-Gilles de Pont-Audemer', *AN* xxxvii (1987), 235–67

Miguet, Michel, *Templiers et hospitaliers en Normandie*, Paris 1995

Miramon, Charles de, *Les 'Donnés' au moyen âge: une forme de vie religieuse laïque v. 1180–v. 1500*, Paris 1999

Mitchell, Piers D., 'An evaluation of the leprosy of King Baldwin IV of Jerusalem in the context of the medieval world', in Bernard Hamilton, *The leper king and his heirs: Baldwin IV and the crusader kingdom of Jerusalem*, Cambridge 2000, 245–58

Molard, F., *Inventaire-sommaire des archives départementales antérieures à 1790: Yonne: archives hospitalières – série H supplément*, iv, Auxerre 1897

Mollat, Michel, *Les Pauvres au moyen âge: étude sociale*, Paris 1978

—— (ed.), *Histoire de Rouen*, Toulouse 1979

Moore, R. I., *The formation of a persecuting society: power and deviance in Western Europe, 950–1250*, Oxford 1987

Mundy, John H., 'Hospitals and leprosaries in twelfth- and early thirteenth-century Toulouse', in John H. Mundy, Richard W. Emery and Benjamin N. Nelson (eds), *Essays in medieval life and thought: presented in honor of Austin Patterson Evans*, New York 1955, 181–205

Murphy, Neil, 'Plague ordinances and the management of infectious diseases in northern French towns, c. 1450–c. 1560', in Clark and Rawcliffe, *The fifteenth century*, xii. 139–59

Musset, Lucien, *Normandie romane*, II: *La Haute-Normandie*, Yonne 1974

—— 'Rouen au temps des Francs et sous les ducs (Ve siècle–1204)', in Mollat, *Histoire de Rouen*, 31–74

Niel, Cécile and Marie-Cécile Truc (with Bruno Penna), 'La Chapelle Saint-Thomas d'Aizier (Eure): premiers résultats de six années de fouille programmée', in Tabuteau, *Étude des lépreux*, 47–107

O'Boyle, Cornelius, *The art of medicine: medical teaching at the University of Paris, 1250–1400*, Leiden 1998

Page, Christopher, 'Music and medicine in the thirteenth century', in Peregrine Horden (ed.), *Music as medicine: the history of music therapy since antiquity*, Aldershot 2000, 109–19

Paresys, Cécile, 'Saint-Ladre de Reims, un cimetière de lépreux?', in Tabuteau, *Étude des lépreux*, 111–22

Peltzer, Jörg, *Canon law, careers and conquest: episcopal elections in Normandy and Greater Anjou, c. 1140–c. 1230*, Cambridge 2008

Periaux, Nicétas, *Dictionnaire indicateur et historique des rues et places de Rouen*, Rouen 1870, repr. Saint-Aubin-les-Elbeuf 1997

Pevsner, Nikolaus, rev. Enid Radcliffe, *The buildings of England: Essex*, Harmondsworth 1965

Peyroux, Catherine, 'The leper's kiss', in Sharon Farmer and Barbara H. Rosenwein (eds), *Monks and nuns, saints and outcasts: religion in medieval society: essays in honor of Lester K. Little*, Ithaca, NY 2000, 172–88

Porquet, Louis, *La Peste en normandie du XIVe au XVIIe siècle*, Vire 1898

Postles, David, 'Monastic burials of non-patronal lay benefactors', *Journal of Ecclesiastical History* xlvii (1996), 620–37

—— 'Lamps, lights and layfolk: "popular" devotion before the Black Death', *Journal of Medieval History* xxv (1999), 97–114

Power, Daniel, 'The French interests of the Marshal earls of Striguil and Pembroke, 1189–1234', ANS xxv (2002), 199–225

—— 'Angevin Normandy', in Christopher Harper-Bill and Elisabeth van Houts (eds), *A companion to the Anglo-Norman world*, Woodbridge 2003, 63–85

—— *The Norman frontier in the twelfth and early thirteenth centuries*, Cambridge 2004

—— 'Rouen and the aristocracy of Angevin Normandy', in Hicks and Brenner, *Society and culture*, 279–308

Rawcliffe, Carole, *Medicine & society in later medieval England*, Stroud 1995

—— 'Learning to love the leper: aspects of institutional charity in Anglo-Norman England', *ANS* xxiii (2000), 231–50

—— *Leprosy in medieval England*, Woodbridge 2006

—— 'Communities of the living and of the dead: hospital confraternities in the later Middle Ages', in Christopher Bonfield, Jonathan Reinarz and Teresa Huguet-Termes (eds), *Hospitals and communities, 1100–1960*, Oxford 2013, 125–54

—— *Urban bodies: communal health in late medieval English towns and cities*, Woodbridge 2013

Richards, Peter, *The medieval leper and his northern heirs*, Cambridge 1977, repr. 2000

Roberts, Charlotte A., 'Conference background and context', in Roberts, Lewis and Manchester, *The past and present of leprosy*, pp. iv–v

—— Mary E. Lewis and Keith Manchester (eds), *The past and present of leprosy: archaeological, historical, palaeopathological and clinical approaches*, Oxford 2002

Roffey, Simon, *Chantry chapels and medieval strategies for the afterlife*, Stroud 2008

——'Medieval leper hospitals in England: an archaeological perspective', *Medieval Archaeology* lvi (2012), 203–33

Ronan, Myles V., 'St Stephen's hospital, Dublin', *Dublin Historical Record* iv (1941–2), 141–8

Rosenwein, Barbara H., *To be the neighbor of Saint Peter: the social meaning of Cluny's property, 909–1049*, Ithaca, NY 1989

Roy, Lyse, *L'Université de Caen aux XVe et XVIe siècles: identité et représentation*, Leiden 2006

Rubin, Miri, *Charity and community in medieval Cambridge*, Cambridge 1987

Sadourny, Alain, 'Des Débuts de la guerre de cent ans à la Harelle', in Mollat, *Histoire de Rouen*, 99–122

—— 'L'Époque communale (1204–début du XIVe siècle)', in Mollat, *Histoire de Rouen*, 75–98

—— 'Les Grandes Familles rouennaises au XIIIe siècle et leur rôle dans la cité', in Bouet and Neveux, *Les Villes normandes*, 267–78

Sanders, I. J., *English baronies: a study of their origin and descent, 1086–1327*, Oxford 1960

Schultz, Michael and Charlotte A. Roberts,, 'Diagnosis of leprosy in skeletons from an English later medieval hospital using histological analysis', in Roberts, Lewis and Manchester, *The past and present of leprosy*, 89–104

Servin, Antoine-Nicolas, *Histoire de la ville de Rouen, capitale du pays et duché de Normandie, depuis sa fondation jusqu'en l'année 1774: suivie d'un essai sur la Normandie littéraire*, Rouen 1775

Six, Manon, 'The burgesses of Rouen in the late twelfth and early thirteenth centuries', in Hicks and Brenner, *Society and culture*, 247–78

Skinner, Patricia, *Women in medieval Italian society, 500–1200*, Harlow 2001

Smith, R. J., 'Henry II's heir: the *acta* and seal of Henry the Young King, 1170–83', *English Historical Review* cxvi (2001), 297–326

Spear, David S., *The personnel of the Norman cathedrals during the ducal period, 911–1204*, London 2006

Stanford, Charlotte A., *Commemorating the dead in late medieval Strasbourg: the cathedral's Book of Donors and its use (1320–1521)*, Farnham 2011

Stratford, Jenny (ed.), *Medieval art, architecture and archaeology at Rouen*, [London] 1993

Stratford, Neil, 'The wall-paintings of the Petit-Quevilly', in Stratford, *Medieval art, architecture and archaeology*, 51–9 and plates

—— 'Le Petit-Quevilly, peintures murales de la chapelle Saint-Julien', in *Congrès Archéologique de France, 161e session 2003: Rouen et Pays de Caux*, Paris 2005, 133–46

Strayer, Joseph R., *The administration of Normandy under Saint Louis*, Cambridge, MA 1932, repr. New York 1971

—— *The royal domain in the bailliage of Rouen*, rev. edn, London 1976

—— *The reign of Philip the Fair*, Princeton, NJ 1980

Sweetinburgh, Sheila, *The role of the hospital in medieval England: gift-giving and the spiritual economy*, Dublin 2004

Tabbagh, Vincent, *Fasti ecclesiae gallicanae: répertoire prosopographique des évêques, dignitaires et chanoines de France de 1200 à 1500*, II: *Diocèse de Rouen*, Turnhout 1998

—— 'L'Exercise de la fonction curiale à Rouen au XVe siècle', in Éric Barré (ed.), *La Paroisse en Normandie au moyen âge: la vie paroissiale, l'église et le cimetière: histoire, art, archéologie*, Saint-Lô 2008, 46–61

Tabuteau, Bruno, 'Combien de lépreux au moyen âge? Essai d'étude quantitative appliquée à la lèpre: les exemples de Rouen et de Bellencombre au XIIIe siècle', *Sources: Travaux historiques* xiii (1988), 19–23

—— 'Histoire et archéologie de la lèpre et des lépreux en Europe et en Méditerranée du moyen âge au temps modernes: 2e table ronde du Groupe de Göttingen', *AN* xlix (1999), 567–600

—— 'Historical research developments on leprosy in France and Western Europe', in Bowers, *The medieval hospital*, 41–56

—— (ed.), *Étude des lépreux et des léproseries au moyen âge dans le nord de la France: histoire – archéologie – patrimoine*, Histoire médiévale et archéologie xx (2007)

Thompson, Kathleen, 'L'Aristocratie anglo-normande et 1204', in Pierre Bouet and Véronique Gazeau (eds), *La Normandie et l'Angleterre au moyen âge*, Caen 2003, 179–87

Touati, François-Olivier, 'Les Léproseries aux XIIème et XIIIème siècles, lieux de conversion?', in Bériou and Touati, *Voluntate dei leprosus*, 1–32

—— *Archives de la lèpre: atlas des léproseries entre Loire et Marne au moyen âge*, Paris 1996

—— *Maladie et société au moyen âge: la lèpre, les lépreux et les léproseries dans la province ecclésiastique de Sens jusqu'au milieu du XIVe siècle*, Brussels 1998

—— 'Contagion and leprosy: myth, ideas and evolution in medieval minds and societies', in Lawrence I. Conrad and Dominik Wujastyk (eds), *Contagion: perspectives from pre-modern societies*, Aldershot 2000, 179–201

—— 'Historiciser la notion de contagion: l'exemple de la lèpre dans les sociétés médiévales', in Sylvie Bazin-Tacchella, Danielle Quéruel and Évelyne

Samama (eds), *Air, miasmes et contagion: les épidémies dans l'antiquité et au moyen âge*, Langres 2001, 157–87

—— 'La Géographie hospitalière médiévale (Orient–Occident, IVe–XVIe siècles): des modèles aux réalités', in Pascal Montaubin (ed.), *Hôpitaux et maladreries au moyen âge: espace et environnement, Histoire médiévale et archéologie* xvii (2004), 7–20

—— '"Aime et fais ce que tu veux": les chanoines réguliers et la revolution de charité au moyen âge', in Michel Parisse (ed.), *Les Chanoines réguliers: émergence et expansion (XIe–XIIIe siècle); actes du sixième colloque international du CERCOR, Le Puy en Velay, 29 juin–1er juillet 2006*, Saint-Étienne 2009, 159–210

VCH, *A history of the county of London*, ed. William Page, London 1909

VCH, *A history of the county of Middlesex*, i, ed. J. S. Cockburn, H. P. F. King and K. G. T. McDonnell, London 1969

Veyrat, Maurice, *Essai chronologique et biographique sur les baillis de Rouen (de 1171 à 1790)*, Rouen 1953

Vincent, Catherine, *Des Charités bien ordonnées: les confréries normandes de la fin du XIIIe siècle au début du XVIe siècle*, Paris 1988

Wallis, Faith (ed.), *Medieval medicine: a reader*, Toronto 2010

Warren, W. L., *Henry II*, London 1973

Westerhof, Danielle, *Death and the noble body in medieval England*, Woodbridge 2008

Wickersheimer, Ernest, *Dictionnaire biographique des médecins en France au moyen âge*, Paris 1936

Yearl, Mary K. K. H., 'Medieval monastic customaries on *minuti* and *infirmi*', in Bowers, *The medieval hospital*, 175–94

Unpublished dissertations etc.

Bonfield, Christopher A., 'The *Regimen sanitatis* and its dissemination in England, c. 1348–1550', PhD, East Anglia 2006

Brenner, Elma, 'Charity in Rouen in the twelfth and thirteenth centuries (with special reference to Mont-aux-Malades)', PhD, Cambridge 2007

Bulot, A., B. Grisel, B. Guillemot and V. Hubert, 'Série H: clergé régulier 17HP à 115HP: abbayes et prieurés: récolement des fonds non classés', unpubl. inventory, ADSM, 1994

Dubois, Catherine, 'Les Rouennais face à la mort au XVe siècle, d'après l'obituaire du prieuré de la Madeleine', MA, Rouen 1990

Everard, Judith A., 'Ralph, son of Stephen' and 'Talbot family', unpubl. notes, Nov. 2005

Madeline, Fanny, 'La Politique de construction des Plantagenêt et la formation d'un territoire politique (1154–1216)', PhD, LAMOP/Université Paris-I 2009

Mesmin, Simone C., 'The leper hospital of Saint Gilles de Pont-Audemer: an edition of its cartulary and an examination of the problem of leprosy in the twelfth and early thirteenth century', PhD, Reading 1978

Poggioli, Peter A., 'From politician to prelate: the career of Walter of Coutances, archbishop of Rouen, 1184–1207', PhD, Johns Hopkins 1984

Rousseau, Louis, 'L'Assistance charitable à Rouen du XIIe au XVIe siècle: l'Hôtel-Dieu de la Madeleine: la police des pauvres', École nationale des Chartes, Paris 1938

Satchell, Max, 'The emergence of leper-houses in medieval England, 1100–1250', D.Phil, Oxford 1998

Six, Manon, '71 H 1–20: fonds des Bernardines de Saint-Aubin de Gournay: répertoire numérique détaillé', unpubl. inventory, ADSM 2008

Tabuteau, Bruno, 'Les Léproseries dans la Seine-Maritime du XIIe au XVe siècle', MA, Rouen 1982

—— 'Une Léproserie normande au moyen âge: le prieuré de Saint-Nicolas d'Évreux du XIIe au XVIe siècle: histoire et corpus des sources', PhD, Rouen 1996

Turner, Victoria, 'Monastic medicine in the visitation records of Eudes Rigaud, archbishop of Rouen (1248–75)', BA, Cambridge 2009

Waldman, Thomas G., 'Hugh "of Amiens", archbishop of Rouen (1130–64)', D.Phil, Oxford 1970

Watson, Sethina C., 'Fundatio, ordinatio and statuta: the statutes and constitutional documents of English hospitals to 1300', D.Phil, Oxford 2004

Yearl, Mary K. K. H., 'The time of bloodletting', PhD, Yale 2005

Index

Names of individuals listed in appendix 2 are not included unless they appear in the main text.

Printed and bound by CPI Group (UK) Ltd, Croydon, CR0 4YY
03/10/2022
03151726-0001